CLASSICS IN
DEVELOPMENTAL MEDICINE
No. 6

(Series Editor: Ross G. Mitchell, M.D.)

———————

PLAY IN CHILDHOOD

by

MARGARET LOWENFELD
M.R.C.S., L.R.C.P.

Psychological Director of
the Institute of Child Psychology
London

———————

With a Foreword by
John Davis

———————

1991
MAC KEITH PRESS

Distributed by
OXFORD: BLACKWELL SCIENTIFIC PUBLICATIONS LTD.
NEW YORK: CAMBRIDGE UNIVERSITY PRESS

First published in this edition 1991

British Library Cataloguing in Publication Data

Lowenfeld, Margaret
    Play in childhood.—2nd ed.—(Classics in developmental medicine, no. 6).
    1. Child psychology
    I. Title II. Series
    155.418

ISBN (UK) 0 901260 84 3
       (USA) 0 521 41331 1

Printed in Great Britain at The Lavenham Press Ltd., Lavenham, Suffolk
Mac Keith Press is supported by **The Spastics Society, London, England**

CONTENTS

FOREWORD

MARGARET LOWENFELD 1890–1973

MARGARET LOWENFELD was in some ways the odd woman out in the set of pioneer child psychiatrists who made London the mecca of their subject before, during and immediately after the second world war—including Melanie Klein, Anna Freud, Donald Winnicott and Susan Isaacs. After a stormy childhood, she qualified in medicine (like her sister, Helena Wright), to become almost immediately involved in relief operations in her father's native Poland, which had been devastated in the fighting that followed the 1914–18 war. This was, not surprisingly, a formative emotional experience which brought home to her the resilience of children under stress and complemented her intellectual training in clinical science. As a research worker she carried out exemplary studies in rheumatic fever and infant nutrition for the Medical Research Council which remain models of their kind. She brought both these elements in her education, as well as her own childhood experiences, to bear on her growing interest in the emotional problems of children, which ultimately led to the establishment of her 'Institute of Child Psychology' in West London, where she adopted an holistic approach to the simultaneous diagnosis and treatment of the children referred to it—making it her particular concern to attend to the cognitive and somatic as well as the affective elements in their developing characters. Her pragmatic approach was in contrast to those who espoused the more theoretical systems of Freud and Klein, but neither did she adopt the medical model with its emphasis on diagnostic categories and its lack of interest in the content of a patient's disturbance.

Though herself a charismatic character who attracted devoted disciples, Lowenfeld professed disbelief in the importance of transference in psychotherapy and put the emphasis on the children themselves being enabled to discover the positive aspects of their personalities. In this context she developed the so-called 'World Technique' for exploring in a semi-structured fashion the important elements in a child's inner world by the way in which he or she arranged a set of representational toy figures in the landscape provided by a tray of sand. For Dr Lowenfeld, playing was the most important way in which children set about ordering their universe as a prelude to the engagements of adult life; and this recognition brought her into conflict with Melanie Klein, for whom it was a symbolic system requiring interpretation in terms of unconscious phantasy. It eventually brought her into alliance with Donald Winnicott who, albeit a disciple of both Freud and Klein, had also come to believe that play is an end in itself for the child.

The world technique was only one of Lowenfeld's inventions for exploring and fostering the abilities of her patients: her Poleidoblocs are still used for teaching the elements of geometry and her Mosaics are even now proving to be a fascinating tool for the exploration of differences in the patterns which different cultures impose on the visual aspects of experience. Yet another insight which Lowenfeld brought to bear on the work of her Institute was the need to integrate bodily activity and rhythmic and gross motor movement into the therapeutic regimen, so as to enable children to become aware of their somatic boundaries and their kinaesthetic experiences—in contrast to the purely verbal methods of the analysts.

But Lowenfeld was not only a gifted practical psychologist, albeit her theoretical position did to some degree lack systematic coherence. Like many of those who fit into Keats' category of the egotistical sublime, she was capable of particular insights into the nature of things—such as her realisation that our awareness of our own state of mind stems from feeling its somatic effects (rather than the latter being caused by the former); and her intellectual friendships with men and women of the calibre of the Oxford philosopher Collingwood and the anthropologist Margaret Mead testify to her quality of mind. She was not a facile writer, however, and her *Play in Childhood* is her only major contribution to the literature on the human nature of children. For this reason alone—as a memorial to a remarkable woman and a way into her manner of thinking and working—it is greatly to be welcomed that Mac Keith Press, who publish *Classics in Developmental Medicine*, have had the perspicacity to re-issue it in their series of seminal texts. It should be pointed out here that what is reproduced is the original first edition and that therefore, sadly in some ways, Margaret Mead's preface and the piece added by Miss M. Kirschner (Lowenfeld's movement therapist) to the second edition are omitted.

Perhaps the time is now ripe for the ecumenical integration of the various psychotherapeutic sects so long devoted to the preservation of particular contributions to our understanding but now ready—as T. S. Eliot put it—to be folded into a single party. Such an eclectic psychotherapy would not ignore the fundamental insights of Klein to the ontological and of Winnicott to the environmental elements in disturbances of character development; but it would also include Lowenfeld's contributions to methodology, her psychosomatic approach to therapy and her recognition of the relationship between cognition and affect. These may have particular relevance to the supposed antinomy between playgroups and nursery education.

JOHN A. DAVIS,
PROFESSOR EMERITUS OF PAEDIATRICS,
UNIVERSITY OF CAMBRIDGE.

PLAY IN CHILDHOOD

FIRST PUBLISHED 1935

PREFACE

THE STANDPOINT from which this book has been written is set out in the Introduction. The materials which have been used are as follows: records made in the Institute of Child Psychology, 26 Warwick Avenue, London, W.9, of the play of children attending that Institute; as wide a reading of published studies of children's play as it has been possible to cover in a life much taken up with private work; and comparison with the experiences of other workers daily in contact with childen, who attended the lecture discussions that form the kernel of this book.

The substance of the chapters that form the bulk of this book was originally given in the spring of 1934 at the Institute of Child Psychology as a series of lecture discussions to an audience consisting of members of H.M. Board of Education, inspectors, principals, and members of training college staffs, headmistresses and staffs of nursery schools. The purpose of the lectures was a discussion of certain conclusions which had been arrived at in regard to the subject of play through a study of the play of children at the Institute, with those whose lives bring them intimately into contact with children who have not shown any form of abnormality. Notes of the discussions will be found throughout the book in footnotes to the appropriate chapters. By this means it was hoped to exclude conclusions deduced entirely from the study of abnormality and to achieve generalisations which apply to the play of children as a whole.

It is interesting to note that the children of whom careful studies have so far been published are children such as would come under consideration of Groups 1–3 of the Introduction, and that these children, as well as those who formed the subject of Professor Piaget's work, and that of Mrs. Isaacs, are all children coming from a selected cultural background. In this sense, they represent to some extent a special class of childhood. The children who form the material of Professor Charlotte Bühler's and Dr. Hildegard Hetzer's studies in Vienna, on the other hand, and those which are the subject of the present study, are children in whom no selection has taken place either of intelligence or of the mentality or cultural background of the parents. Owing to the general economic situation of this country in 1928–34, and to the fact that children admitted to the Institute are accepted on an economic basis, although the main bulk of the children are those who attend the elementary schools, children coming from homes with a cultured background have also been included. At all points, the experience gained from observation of these children has been compared and collated with experience of children seen in private practice, and no significant difference between the groups has been found. Details concerning the type of children studied, methods of study, etc., will be found in Chapter II.

It remains for me to extend my very sincere thanks to the whole staff of the Institute for their never-failing generosity and help in the preparation of the manuscript, and to Mr. Norman Cliff for steady counsel, criticism, and consistent help in the revision of the text. I especially wish to thank Mr. Clifford Sully and Messrs. Longmans, Green & Co. Ltd. for kind permission to quote from Professor James Sully's *Studies of Childhood*; Messrs. D. Appleton-Century Company Inc., London and New York, for their generous permission for rather extensive quotations from *Aspects of Child Life and Education*, and *Youth: Its Education, Regimen and Hygiene* by G. Stanley Hall; Messrs. Heinemann Ltd. for permission to quote from *The Play of Man* by Karl Groos; Mr. Douglas Byng and Messrs. John Lane, The Bodley Head Ltd., for their courtesy in permitting me to quote from *The Byng Ballads*; Mrs. Drage for permission to reproduce part of her book *Una Mary*; Dr. Charlotte Bühler for her kindness in allowing quotations from *Kindheit und Jugend*, *The First Year of Life*, *The Social Behaviour of the Child*, and *The Child and its Activity with Practical Material*; and Dr. Susan Isaacs for very kindly permitting me to include quotations from *Intellectual Growth in Young Children* and *Social Development in Young Children* for comparison with my records. I wish also to thank very warmly my colleague, Dr. Ethel Dukes, for help in reading the manuscript, and Miss Brownsmith, Mrs. Brown, Mr. P. I. Painter and Dr. Lotte Danzinger for help with the Bibliography.

21 DEVONSHIRE PLACE,
  LONDON, W.

INTRODUCTION

THERE IS hardly any feature of human life to which so little serious consideration has been given as that of children's play. The present study is offered to the reader because of the writer's belief that there is a connection between the play of children and the life of adult man, and that in this little-regarded aspect of the life of the juvenile fraction of humanity can be found clues to some of the most perplexing puzzles that face adult man in his relationships to his fellows.

One of the curious features of the modern world is the contrast between our enormously increased power to control the forces of nature, and our failure to enjoy the fruits of this power through inability to control intelligently our own corporate actions.

It is not credible that there should be another source for our actions than ourselves, yet the perplexing fact remains that what we corporately wish to do we do not, and that which we earnestly desire to hinder we find ourselves inevitably bringing about.

Our increased control over nature seems to be exactly balanced by an increasing bewilderment about ourselves. Unconquered, however, in the face of this paradox, the human mind refuses to admit defeat, and from the darkest aspects of its peril begins to forge new weapons of attack.

Every one of the great battles the human mind wages with its universe h is had its beginning in the urgent pressure arising from some clamant need. Since happiness is a state of passive enjoyment, it does not give rise to such pressing enquiries as " Why? " and " Wherefore? " Out of acute discomfort alone do such questions arise. It is, therefore, natural and inevitable that the first impetus towards man's new knowledge of himself should come from the pressure of mental despair and disease.

Seeds germinate in the dark, and it is in semi-darkness that this battle begins, the darkness both of mental misery and of our own ignorance.

The field is so vast and our knowledge of it is so infinitesimal that an attack at practically any point may yield the most valuable results. Modern work in dynamic psychology has given indications that in the study of children clues may be found to laws of general significance that may not be attainable in any other way; and it is such a belief that lies behind this study of childhood play.

.   .   .   .

To a primitive society young people are important in three ways—they are a relaxation from toil, an earnest of future strength to the tribe, and as they grow to marriageable age they become the focus of the economic cares and ambitions of the family.

In very primitive societies, where a child must rely upon itself* for protection from danger, adults devote a great deal of time to play with their young.[1,2]

In more developed societies, where the protection of children is undertaken by society at large, the tendency is for the child to pass into the background of social living and to take on social importance again only at puberty.† Life at this stage is no longer lived hand in hand with the danger of annihilation, and there is, as it were, a long pause for each child after birth until the curtain goes up again on adolescence. This period is devoted to education, and during its sway children cease to be regarded as important members of the community, and are considered rather as the irrational and immature larvæ of potential adults. The whole significance of the child at this stage lies in its progress towards becoming a successful adult.

With the further development of civilisation and the achievement of comparative safety for the adult, this exclusive concentration of the grown-up mind upon the developmental aspect of childhood slowly changes, and once more, as in very primitive stages of society, the child as a child becomes an object of interest. With the achievement of relative peace and plenty, the extraordinary differences between the behaviour of children and of adults strike upon the adult mind, and out of the wonder that is aroused by them the scientific study of children as children arises.

Any worker in this field finds himself at the outset faced with a double obstacle. The material of his study is at once too familiar and too unknown. It is as if a man seeking literature were to find himself suddenly in an attractive library of reasonable size and easy accessibility, but stocked with books written in a language incomprehensible to him. The rules which govern adult thought and behaviour do not influence children. How then are such behaviour and thoughts to be understood? Hitherto the answer given has run something like this: "The child is the potential adult. Let us study him, then, from that point of view."

From the beginning of the serious study of childhood, the work that has been done can be separated into four groups‡:

*[Editor's note: Dr Lowenfeld uses the pronouns 'it' and 'he' interchangeably to denote a child of unspecified sex and 'she' only when a female child is specifically mentioned. While it is recognised that this may offend the sensibilities of some modern readers, no attempt has been made to change her usage.]

†For example, note the extensive practice of infanticide by which the Greek and Roman world controlled its population and the innumerable losses of children by disease and death in Europe in the Middle Ages.

‡Details of the books to which reference is made under each section will be found in the bibliography at the end of the Introduction.

1. *Personal studies of children by their parents or relatives.*

Perhaps the best-known examples of this group are the study by Preyer of his little boy, and by Dr. and Mrs. Stern of their own children. To these should be added the study by Miss Shinn of her niece Ruth, that of his daughter Roswitha by Otto Ernst, of his son by Darwin, and the diaries of Ernst and Gertrud Scupin concerning their son Bubi. Into this group should come also those portions of autobiographies that give valuable information about certain aspects of childhood.

2. *Studies of the processes of development in children from birth to maturity.*

In this group fall the work of Charlotte Bühler, of Baldwin and of Gesell, and the many independent studies that have been made of a child's first year of life. This group can be divided as follows:

(*a*) *Studies of the evolution of the senses, of the motor capacities and of eye-hand co-ordination.* An excellent bibliography for those interested in this aspect of child study will be found in the *Handbook of Child Psychology* (Oxford Univ. Press, 1931).

(*b*) *Studies of the physiological functions in childhood*—growth, sleep, smiling, eating, excretion—both normal and abnormal. Here the work of Baldwin, Descœudres, Blatz, and many others comes to mind.

(*c*) *Studies of the development of language in children.* There is a very large literature in relation to this section, some indication of which will be found in the bibliography at the end of this Introduction.

(*d*) *Studies of processes of intellectual development in the child and the adolescent.* It is impossible to do more than indicate (as is attempted in the list of references at the end of this Introduction) the mass of material that confronts the observer on this aspect of child life, including, as it does, all problems of learning and of pedagogy. The whole of the problems of education and those investigations upon which education is based come under this heading.

3. *Studies of the emotional reactions of children.*

In relation to this aspect, it is clear that methods of investigation of emotion and behaviour which are applicable to the adult cannot be used with a child, and new methods have to be devised. Hitherto investigation has proceeded upon five lines:

(*a*) Study of children in test circumstances.
(*b*) Study of the reactions of children in their normal surroundings.
(*c*) Study of the behaviour of children in comparison with the behaviour of apes and other animals.
(*d*) Study of the behaviour of children in comparison with that of

primitive peoples.

(e) Studies of the social behaviour of children.

Under section (a) come those series of tests which set a child in the midst of strictly controlled experimental conditions to which his reactions can be noted. From statistical correlations of the results thus obtained it is hoped that natural laws of development may be deduced.

In the view of those whose work is collected under section (b) the arbitrariness of the tests used in section (a) greatly detracts from their value. The contention put forward by workers in this section is that the nature of childhood is such that its behaviour is *altered* by "standardised" conditions, and that standard tests of this kind do not test normal behaviour. The observations that are made by workers in section (b), in contrast to those of the previous section, are carried out in the ordinary surroundings of the children's lives. Incidents normal to a child's ordinary life are selected for use as tests, and the results obtained are compared with each other in the attempt to create standards of development.

The rise of the evolutionary theory of the development of man brought as its natural corollary the perception that man shares with many other animals, particularly apes, certain common features. Animals have long been used for experiment in the study of adult physiological processes, and it is logical that the same type of comparisons should now be made for behaviour. The work of Koffka, to quote only one example, has shown how much illumination can be drawn from such work.

Anthropological study of primitive peoples shows them to be in outlook and behaviour in many ways like the children of civilised communities. It is natural therefore that we should turn to studies of the lives of primitive peoples for light upon the problems of childish forms of behaviour.

The three aspects of study so far considered have taken as their norm for comparison the average, reasonably intelligent, reasonably successful child or adult, and have deliberately endeavoured to confine attention to what might fairly be taken as the normal or the expected in childhood. This is by no means the only aspect of childhood. That group of workers interested in child maladjustment in U.S.A. and in Europe have, on the other hand, selected for study and treatment children who show a *deviation* from the norm.

We come, therefore, to the work of another group.

4. *Studies of abnormal behaviour in children.*

By the workers in this group, children are in the main regarded from three angles:

(a) *As members of society.* Under this heading would come the work of Adler, of the Child Guidance group, and such work of Jung as touches children.

(*b*) *As examples of physiological law.* The chief exponent of this school is Professor Watson.

(*c*) *As individuals showing an unsuccessful personal development.* Here should be included the work of all child psycho-therapists, that of the Institute of Child Psychology, and of the child psycho-analysts.

It would seem strange, in surveying so exhaustive a list of angles of study, to suggest that any serious aspect of the subject can exist to which consideration has not already been very extensively given.

But there is one characteristic which runs throughout the work which has previously been cited. Each aspect, however greatly differing from its neighbour, shares with it a common characteristic in that each is essentially an investigation into the rate and mode of development in children of qualities which are characteristic of, and perfectly manifested by, adult cultural beings. Studies of apes and of primitive human beings, in so far as they have reference to child psychology, have had as their motive a search for the light that they may throw upon the development of civilised man.

That is to say, the problem the investigator has put to himself throughout all this work has been, " At what point in the evolution of a human being, and in what shape, does this or that adult characteristic (see Groups 1–3) appear? And what are the paths followed in its development from that moment to the appearance of the standard adult version of that quality? " This question is supplemented by the parallel enquiry, as in the work of Jaensch, of Peters, and of Busemann, as to "how much variation do different children show in this development, and of what nature is this variation? "

On the other hand, workers in Group 4, among whom the writer is one, put to themselves another problem, which may be stated as: " How exactly does this particular child *deviate* from normal development or behaviour, and what is the cause of this deviation? "

In all these enquiries, adult behaviour is taken as the norm, and the child is seen always in relation to that norm as a creature of shifting powers and changing reality.

Modern dynamic psychology, however, has suggested that certain of the elements of a child's nature and outlook do *not* change, in the process of growth, into adult versions of those elements, but persist unchanged in some part of the mind and form the ultimate background to all adult life.

If this be so, then the behaviour and thoughts of children are not, as we have so far assumed, essentially immature, worthy only of passing attention, but become rather of essential significance, since in them are to be found clues for the understanding of certain features of adult human nature.

This, if true, is a challenging thought, and sets childhood in a light in which as a whole we are unaccustomed to seeing it. The life of the child, from being regarded as a thing of beauty or of inconsequence, comes to reveal itself as pregnant with greater issues; and the mind of the child to hold within itself clues to the understanding of corporate humanity.

If this be true, we shall expect to find in certain aspects of childhood, not larval stages of ultimate growth, but an actual mirror of certain aspects of adult behaviour.

This is the situation presented in the study of the nature of children's play. From being a charming embroidery upon the normal purpose of man, conceived as growth and learning, the nature of play comes instead to occupy a prominent place in the problems of mankind.

Play is a phenomenon peculiarly characteristic of the young. In contrast to the whole range of other faculties in life, it steadily diminishes in frequency and importance with developing years, until some adult lives are entirely devoid of any play element whatever. If there is, therefore, any element of childhood that is of permanent significance, it is logical to expect that the clearest evidence of it will be found somewhere in relation to play.

The chapters that follow are a study of children's play, and an attempt to indicate some of the mechanisms out of which the impulse to play arises.

The classifications into which the forms of play in this book have been divided have been arrived at through study of play itself and not from *a priori* conceptions derived from other work. An attempt has been made at each point to select illustrative notes from the records of children observed at the Institute of Child Psychology, which bring into relief the form of play described in the text. In each case the initials, age, and sex of the child have been given, and for purposes of comparison, also to illustrate the variety of forms of play that any one child may show, many examples have been included from the same children.

Play in childhood is an exceedingly complex phenomenon. It is an activity which combines into a single whole very diverse strands of thought and experience. Many of these persist in adult life. For example, in the *Byng Ballads*[3], written for adult amusement, there appear the following verses:

> *My favourite charger threw me*
> *In a cesspool on a farm*
> *A whip said, " Now they've lost the scent.*
> *Why do these things occur? "*
> *I said, " I think I've found it,*
> *And it isn't Quelques-fleurs! "*
>   *Ta-rah! Ta-rah!*
> *Tantivy! Tantivy! Whoops!*

> *When my throat went so dry shouting out " Ship ahoys,"*
> *To a boat sailing by I just cried, " Hullo, boys! "*
> *But the only reply was a very rude noise,*
> *Oh! I'm well on the rocks, and I know it.*

The same themes will be found in the play of R.L. on page 75, exploited as jokes by a boy of six. It may be objected that this is not a very desirable part of human nature, but the reply is that if any answer is to be found to the riddle of human behaviour, all forms of behaviour must be taken into account. It is the author's contention that the mechanisms of play do not entirely disappear with the ending of childhood, but that many of them show a tendency to survive and to motivate also certain aspects of adult life.

Chapter I of this book is devoted to an historical account of theories of the meaning of children's play, and Chapter II to a discussion of the difficulties which attend any attempt to study children at play.

Activity as a mainspring of play animates both men and animals, and a study of play as movement will be found in Chapter III.

The primitive impulses and desires that provoke rhymes of the kind just quoted are common to many forms of play, and are considered in Chapter IV.

Maeterlinck's *Bluebird*[4] and Kenneth Grahame's *Wind in the Willows*[5] are adult dramatisations of ideas of phantasy that come from time to time to many gifted minds. Chapter V is a study of children's versions of the same activity.

Every adult has at some time to come to terms with the reality that surrounds him. No individual can comprehend even a tenth part of the phenomena he daily meets, and without the help of literature and the drama even that tenth would be beyond his power. The ordinary man in these days relies for his picture of the meaning of the events he sees around him, as A. P. Herbert has so delightfully illustrated in the *Water Gipsies*[6], on the novelist, the dramatist, and the scenario writer, for functions which, in earlier days, were performed by scriptural writings, ballads, and heroic stories. This necessity of the human mind to dramatise these elements of its environment that it perceives, in order to be able emotionally to assimilate them, is a characteristic that runs throughout the whole fabric of human life. In childhood it begins first as the type of play illustrated in Chapter VI. Realism, romance, and satire all find their beginning in the play of children and in the child's play-relation to its environment. Examples of each rudimentary form of art will be found in the play of the children we are reviewing.

Play as a preparation for life is a mechanism peculiar to infancy; it forms the great link between man and animals. It is the characteristic that appears most strongly in the play of animals. Chapter VII is a consideration of play from this angle.

Among certain races, such as the Anglo-Saxons, group games remain popular throughout life, and the reasons given in Chapter VIII for the failure of certain children to join in games apply also to adult members of these races who are similarly placed.

Perhaps there is nothing in which the kinship of child and adult stands out more clearly, or in which the persistence of " childish " traits in adults can be more vividly seen, than in buffoonery. All the world loves a clown, and in the great Christmas circuses the clown's fooling evokes as sure a response from adults as from the children they have accompanied. There are many causes and kinds of laughter, and in Chapter IX will be found a discussion of their varieties.

Leaving altogether on one side the question of group games, some children are unable to play at all, just as some adults throughout their lives are unable to mix socially. Chapter X discusses the elements that go to make up this situation, and the kinds of children in which this form of behaviour can be found. It is too early as yet to say how fixed are these mechanisms of behaviour, but some of these types are persistent, and adult lives will show as many and as clear examples of them as childhood.

Finally, in Chapter XI will be found a summary of the author's views in regard to the nature of play and the place that it takes in the general development of man. In the Appendix will be found an example too long to include properly within the subject matter of this book, and yet itself of considerable interest.

BIBLIOGRAPHY TO INTRODUCTION

SECTION 1 (page 4)

DARWIN, C.   'Biographical sketch of an infant.' *Mind*, 1877, **2**, 285–294.

ERNST, O.   *Roswitha's Day.* (Translated by Caton, A. C.) London: A. C. Caton, 1913.

Roswitha or Philosophy? (Translated by Caton, A. C.) London: A. C. Caton, 1914.

HALL, W. S.   'The first five hundred days of a child's life. V.' *Child Studies*, 1897, **2**, 586–608.

HOGAN, L. E.   *A Study of a Child.* New York: Harper, 1898.

PREYER, W.   *Die geistige Entwickling in der ersten Kindheit.* Stuttgart: Union, 1893.

Mental Development in the Child. (Translated by Brown, H. W.) New York: Appleton, 1893.

SCUPIN, E., SCUPIN, G.   *Bubi's erste Kindheit.* Leipzig: Grieben, 1907.

SHARP, E.   *The Child Grows Up.* London: John Lane, Bodley Head, 1929.

SHINN, M. W.   *Notes on the Development of a Child.* Berkeley: University of California Publications, 1893–1899.

Biography of a Baby. Boston: Houghton Mifflin, 1900.

STERN, W.   *Psychologie der frühen Kindheit, bis zum sechsten Lebensjahre.* Leipzig: Quelle und Meyer, 1914.

Psychology of Early Childhood, up to the Sixth Year of Age. (Translated from the 3rd Edn. by Barwell, A.) New York: Holt, 1924.

STERN W., STERN C.   *Erinnerung, Aussage und Lüge in der ersten Kindheit. Monographie über die seelische Entwicklung des Kindes, II.* Leipzig: Barth, 1909.

WOOLLEY, H. T.   *Agnes: a Dominant Personality in the Making. Pedagogical Seminary and Journal of Genetic Psychology*, 1925, **32** (4).

SECTION 2 (page 4)

GENERAL

ARLITT, A. H.   *Psychology of Infancy and Early Childhood.* London and New York: McGraw-Hill, 1930.

BALDWIN, B. T., STECHER, L. I.   *The Psychology of the Pre-school Child.* New York: Appleton, 1924.

BLANTON, M. G.   'The behaviour of the human infant during the first thirty days of life.' *Psychological Reviews* 1917, **24**, 456–483.

BÜHLER, C.   *Kindheit und Jugend: Genese des Bewusstseins. Psychologische Monographien, Vol. III.* Leipzig: Hirzel, 1928.

The First Year of Life. (Translated by Greenberg, P., Ripin, R.) New York: John Day, 1930.

From Birth to Maturity. London: Kegan Paul, 1935.

BURR, C. W.   'The reflexes in early infancy.' *American Journal of Diseases of Children*, 1921, 21, 529–533.

de ANGELIS, F.   'Reflexes of the new-born.' *American Journal of Diseases of Children*, 1923, **26**, 211–215.

DESCŒUDRES, A.   *Le Développement de l'Enfant de Deux à Sept Ans.* Neuchâtel and Paris: Delachaux & Niestlé, 1921.

FREUD, S.   'Infantile sexuality.' *In: Three Contributions to the Theory of Sex.* New York and Washington: Nervous and Mental Diseases Publishing Co., 1930.

GESELL, A.   *Infancy and Human Growth.* New York: Macmillan, 1928.

PEREZ, B.   *La Psychologie de l'Enfant: les Trois Premières Années.* Paris: Alcan, 1878.

The First Three Years of Childhood. (Edited and translated by Christie, A. M.) Chicago: Marquis, 1885.

SECTION 2 (a) (page 4)

ANDERSON, J. E.   'The development of motor, linguistic and intellectual skills in young children.' *In: Report of the Third Conference on Research in Child Development. Part I. Critical Reviews.* Washington D.C.: National Research Council, 1929.

BRACE, D. K.   *Measuring Motor Ability: a Scale of Motor Ability Tests.* New York: Barnes, 1927.

BRIAN, C. R., GOODENOUGH, F. L.   'The relative potency of color and form perception at various ages.' *Journal of Experimental Psychology*, 1929, **12**, 197–213.

BRYAN, W. L.   'On the development of voluntary motor ability.' *American Journal of Psychology*, 1892, **5**, 125–205.

DEARBORN, G. V. N.   *Moto-sensory Development: Observations on the First Three Years of a Child.* Baltimore: Warwick & York, 1910.

OJEMANN, R. H.   'Studies in handedness: I. A technique for testing unimanual handedness'; 'II. Testing bimanual handedness.' *Journal of Educational Psychology*, 1930, **21**, 597–611; 695–702.

PEAR, T. H.   *Skill in Work and Play.* London: Metheun, 1924.

WELLMAN, B. — *The Development of Motor Co-ordination in Young Children: an Experimental Study in the Control of Hand and Arm Movements. University of Iowa Studies in Child Welfare Vol. 3, No. 2. 1926.*

SECTION 2 (*b*) (page 4)

BALDWIN, B. T. — *Physical Growth of Children from Birth to Maturity. University of Iowa Studies in Child Welfare, Vol. 1, No. 1. 1921.*

Weight-height-age Standards (nude) in Metric Units for American-born Boys (Girls) of School Age. Iowa City: Iowa Child Welfare Research Station, 1924.

BLATZ, W. E., CHANT, M. — 'A study of sleeping habits of children.' *Genetic Psychology Monographs*, 1928, **4**, 13–43.

BURNHAM, W. H. — 'The hygiene of sleep.' *Pediatric Seminars*, 1920, **27**, 1–35.

DAVIS, C. — 'Self selection of diet by newly weaned infants.' *American Journal of Diseases of Children*, 1928, **36**, 651–679.

DESCŒUDRES, A. — (See Section 2, General.)

GAUGER, M. E. — *Modifiability of Response to Taste Stimuli in the Pre-school Child.* Columbia University Contributions to Education, No. 348. 1929.

KATZ, D. — 'Psychologische Probleme des Hungers und Appetits, insbesondere beim Kinde.' *Zeitschrift für Kinderforschule*, 1928, **34**, 158–197.

SCAMMON, R. E. — 'The measurement and analysis of human growth.' *In: Report of the Third Conference on Research in Child Development.* Washington D.C.: National Research Council, 1929.

TERMAN, L. M., HOCKING, A. — 'The sleep of school children: its distribution according to age and its relation to physical and mental efficiency.' *Journal of Educational Psychology*, 1913, **4**, 138–147.

WASHBURN, R. W. — 'A study of the smiling and laughing of infants in the first year of life.' *Genetic Psychology Monographs*, 1929, **6**, 397–537.

WEST, G. M. — 'The growth of the human body.' *Educational Review*, 1896, **12**, 284–289.

SECTION 2 (*c*) (page 4)

BÜHLER, K. — *Die geistige Entwicklung des Kindes.* Jena: Fischer, 1918.

PIAGET, J. — *Le Langage et la Pensée chez l'Enfant.* Neuchâtel and Paris: Delachaux & Niestlé, 1923.

The Language and Thought of the Child. (Translated by Warden, M.) London: Kegan Paul; New York: Harcourt Brace, 1926.

Le Jugement et le Raisonnement chez l'Enfant. Neuchâtel and Paris: Delachaux & Niestlé, 1924.

Judgement and Reasoning in the Child. (Translated by Warden, M.) London: Kegan Paul; New York: Harcourt Brace, 1928.

La Représentation du Monde chez l'Enfant. Paris: Alcan, 1926.

The Child's Conception of the World. (Translated by Tomlinson, J., Tomlinson, A.) London: Kegan Paul; New York: Harcourt Brace, 1929.

SECTION 2 (*d*) (page 4)

GESELL, A. *The Mental Growth of the Pre-school Child: a Psychological Outline of Normal Development from Birth to the Sixth Year.* New York: Macmillan, 1925.

HOLLINGWORTH, L. S. *Gifted Children: their Nature and Nurture.* New York: Macmillan, 1926.

ISAACS, S. *Intellectual Growth in Young Children.* London: Routledge; New York: Harcourt Brace, 1930.

JOHNSON, B. J. *Mental Growth of Children in Relation to Rate of Growth in Bodily Development.* New York: Dutton, 1925.

SECTION 3 (*a*) (page 4)

BECHTEREW, W. *Über die individuelle Entwicklung der neuropsychischen Spare nach den Ergebnissen der objektiven Psychologie.* Westnik Psychologii, 1910.

Über die Entwicklung der neuropsychischen Tätigkeit im ersten Halbjahre des kindlichen Lebens. Westnik Psychologii, 1912.

Neues in der Reflextheorie und Physiologie des Nervensystems. 1925.

GESELL, A. (See previous section.)

SECTION 3 (*b*) (page 4)

BÜHLER, C. (See previous sections. Also *Veröffentlichungen des psychologischen Instituts der Universität Wien seit dem Jahre 1924.*)

SECTION 3 (*c*) (page 4)

KOFFKA, K. *The Growth of the Mind: an Introduction to Child Psychology.* (Translated by Ogden, R. M.) London: Kegan Paul; New York: Harcourt Brace, 1924.

KÖHLER, W. *The Mentality of Apes.* (Translated by Winter, E.) New York: Harcourt Brace, 1925.

THORNDIKE, E. L.   *Animal Intelligence.* New York: Macmillan, 1911.

SECTION 3 (*d*) (page 4)

HAMBLY, W. D.   *Origins of Education among Primitive Peoples: a Comparative Study in Racial Development.* London: Macmillan, 1926.

KIDD, D.   *Savage Childhood: a Study of Kafir Children.* London: Black, 1906.

MALINOWSKI, B.   *Sex and Repression in Savage Society.* London: Kegan Paul; New York: Harcourt Brace, 1927.

MEAD, M.   *Coming of Age in Samoa.* New York: Morrow, 1928.

Growing up in New Guinea. New York: Morrow, 1930. (London: Kegan Paul, 1931.)

'The primitive child.' *In:* Murchison, C. (Ed.) *A Handbook of Child Psychology.* London: Oxford University Press; Worcester, MA: Clark University Press, 1931.

MILLER, N.   *The Child in Primitive Society.* New York: Brentano's, 1928.

VAN WATERS, M.   'The adolescent girl among primitive peoples.' *Journal of Religious Psychology,* 1913, **6**, 375–421; 1914, **7**, 75–120.

SECTION 3 (*e*) (page 5)

BRIDGES, K. M. B.   *Social and Emotional Development of the Pre-school Child.* London: Kegan Paul, 1931.

ISAACS, S.   *Social Development in Young Children. A Study of Beginnings.* London: Routledge; New York: Harcourt Brace, 1933.

SECTION 4 (*a*) (page 5)

ADLER, A.   *Heilen und Bilden.* Munich: J. Bergmann, 1922.

The Practice and Theory of Individual Psychology. (Translated by Radin, P.) London: Kegan Paul, 1924.

STEVENSON, G. S., SMITH, G.   *Child Guidance Clinics: a Quarter Century of Development.* London: Oxford University Press; New York: The Commonwealth Fund, 1934.

WICKES, F. G.   *The Inner World of Childhood: a Study in Analytical Psychology.* London and New York: Appleton, 1927.

SECTION 4 (*b*) (page 6)

WATSON, J. B.   *Behaviorism.* New York: People's Institute Publishing Co., 1924.

WATSON, J. B., WATSON, R. R.   'Studies in infant psychology.' *Scientific Monthly,* 1921, **13**, 493–515.

SECTION 4 (*c*) (page 6)

CAMERON, H.   *The Nervous Child. 3rd Edn.* London: Oxford University Press, 1925.

NEILL, A. S.   *The Problem Child.* London: Herbert Jenkins, 1926.

FLÜGEL, J. C.   *The Psycho-analytic Study of the Family.* London: Hogarth Press, 1921.

FREUD, S.   'Analyse der Phobie eines 5-jährigen Knaben.' *In:* Abraham, K., Hitchman, E. (Eds.) *Jahrbuch für Psychoanalyse und Psychopathologie, Vol. I.* Leipzig and Vienna: Deuticke, 1909.

'Analysis of a phobia in a five-year-old boy.' *In: Collected Papers, Vol. 3.* London: Hogarth Press, 1925.

Drei Abhandlungen zur Sexualtheorie, 2nd Edn. Leipzig and Vienna: Deuticke, 1910.

Three Contributions to the Theory of Sex. Nervous and Mental Disease Monograph Series, No. 7. (Translated by Brill, A. A.) 1930.

HUG-HELLMUTH, H. V.   'On the technique of child analysis.' (Translated by Gabler, R., Low, B.) *International Journal of Psychoanalysis,* 1921, **2**, 287–305.

KLEIN, M.   *Die Psychoanalyse des Kindes.* Vienna: Internationaler Psychoanalytischer Verlag, 1932.

The Psychoanalysis of Children. (Translated by Strachey, A.) London Hogarth Press and Institute of Psychoanalysis, 1932.

SCHMIDEBERG, M.   'Psychoneuroses of childhood: their etiology and treatment.' *British Journal of Medical Psychology,* 1933, **13**, 313–327.

'The play-analysis of a three-year-old girl.' *International Journal of Psycho-analysis,* 1934, **15**, 245–264.

'The psycho-analysis of asocial children and adolescents.' *International Journal of Psycho-analysis,* 1935, **16**, 22–48.

SEARL, M. N.   'Some analytical illustrations from a child's behaviour.' *International Journal of Psycho-analysis,* 1924, **5**, 358–362.

'Symposium on child analysis.' *International Journal of Psycho-analysis,* 1927, **8**, 377–380.

'The rôles of ego and libido in development.' *International Journal of Psycho-analysis,* 1930, **11**, 125–149.

'Play, reality and aggression.' *International Journal of Psycho-analysis,* 1933, **14**, 310–320.

'A note on symbols and early intellectual activity.'
International Journal of Psycho-analysis, 1933, **14**, 391–397.

FREUD, A.
Einfürung in die Technik der Kinder-analyse. Leipzig, Vienna and Zurich: Internationaler Psychoanalytischer Verlag, 1925.
Introduction to the Technique of Child Analysis. Nervous and Mental Diseases Monograph Series, No. 48. (Translated by Clark, L. P.) New York: Nervous and Mental Diseases Publishing Co., 1928.

LOWENFELD, M.
'A new approach to the problem of psychoneurosis in childhood.' *British Journal of Medical Psychology*, 1931, **11**, 194–227.
'Psychogenic factors in chronic disease in childhood.' *Medical Women's Federation Newsletter*, July 1934.

BUSEMANN, A.
Die Jugend im eigenen Urteil: eine Untersuchung zur Jugendkunde. Langensalze: Beltz, 1926.

JAENSCH, E. R.
Eidetic Imagery and Typological Methods of Investigation. (Translated by Oeser, O.) London: Kegan Paul, 1930.

KLÜVER, H.
'Studies on the eidetic type and on eidetic imagery.' *Psychological Bulletin*, 1928, **25**, 69–104.

PETERS, W.
'Zur psychologischen Typik des abnormen Kindes.' *Zeitschrift für pädiatrische Psychologie*, 1927, **28**, 19–35.

CHAPTER I

HISTORICAL THEORIES OF PLAY

Sir Sampson: Did you come a volunteer into the world? or did I, with the lawful authority of a parent, press you to the service?
Valentine: I know no more why I came, than you do why you called me. But here I am . . . I am of myself, a plain, easy, simple creature; and to be kept at small expense: but the retinue that you gave me are craving and invincible; they are so many devils you have raised, and will have employment.

WILLIAM CONGREVE.
Love for Love, Act II, scene vii. Dialogue between Sir Sampson Ledgend and his son Valentine.

So MUCH AMBIGUITY has arisen from time to time over the use of the word "play", as also over the exact interpretation of the word "child", that before any useful examination can be made either of play itself, or of matters concerning a child or children, some agreement must be arrived at as to the sense in which either word is used.

As regards the word "child", it has during the history of the English language born very many meanings, and in this book will be taken as embracing the years between eighteen months (early toddler) and early adolescence—that is to say, the period covered by the nursery school and ordinary school years of the elementary school child.*

An equivalent term to the English word "play" is to be found in all European languages. In each language the meaning of the word "play", like that of the word "child", has shown great flexibility. In the *Oxford English Dictionary*, among the very large number of meanings given, the following groups may be distinguished: Play as free activity or movement in general; play as the carrying out of something which is not to be taken seriously, but is done merely in sport or frolic; to engage in a game, to play it; to perform dramatically, and, with the derived sense, to represent in mimic action, to play out; to play on musical instruments.

In the study of children's play each and every form of meaning will be found to be implied.

*It should be noted that the age which marks the end of school for the elementary school child is the beginning of the serious education of the public school boy and girl.

Children have played since the dawn of civilisation, and descriptions of their games are to be found throughout the literature of mankind. Every civilisation has handed on to its children, from one generation to another, traditional types of games.[7] Moreover, in reference to children, it is in this sense that to the present day the word "play" is most generally used.

Since all activities of children other than lessons, eating, and sleeping seem to the watching adult to have no serious purpose, a description of them as play appears apt and fitting, and to draw a line rigidly, for example, between the play of an individual playing alone, and games which are played in groups, seems the act of a purist.

It was Froebel who, in the early part of last century, first pointed out that the games that children play in groups to set rules are only part, and a very small part, of the total play life of children, and that play in itself in children is not *relaxation*, but the most significant aspect of childhood.

"Play," said Froebel[8], "then, is the highest expression of human development in childhood, for it alone is the free expression of what is in the child's soul. It is the purest and most spiritual product of the child, and at the same time it is a type and copy of human life at all stages and in all relations. . . For to one who has insight into human nature, the trend of the whole future life of the child is revealed in his freely chosen play."

It was Froebel's genius to have discovered play as the appropriate vehicle and helpmate of education. Primarily an educationalist with his whole mind and heart centred in education, he was at the same time an amazingly intuitive, acute, and sympathetic observer of children. Throughout his writings illuminating remarks are scattered, almost as if by chance, on the varieties and significance of play, but at no point does he attempt a systematic classification of children's play as play.

Towards the end of the nineteenth century, Spencer[9] put forward the theory that children's play arises out of the discharge of an excess of energy in the brain centres in childhood, and the child plays because he has a superabundant supply of energy.

In 1884 Grasberger[10] remarked that hitherto no satisfactory classification of play had been made, and in 1896 Professor Karl Groos published the first scientific study of the *Play of Animals*[11], which was followed a few years later by his book on the *Play of Man*[12]. At about the same time, working in America, Stanley Hall and his colleagues had begun to put out a series of papers that were systematic and painstaking studies of various aspects of child life, and which were afterwards collected into *Aspects of Child Life and Education*[13] and *Youth: Its Education, Regimen, and Hygiene*[14]. In England, Sully, then Professor of Psychology at University College, London, published in 1896 his *Studies of Childhood*.

Groos, working from a theory which links the play of childhood with the play of animals, grouped play into seven major and sixty minor varieties. He regarded play as the expression of instinct, and particularly of that form of instinct which impels animals to train themselves in infancy for the rôles they are to play in maturity.

Stanley Hall, on the other hand, writing between 1896 and 1904, takes the view that in play the child epitomises and recapitulates the progress of the race.

"True play", he writes, "never practices what is phyletically new. . . . I regard play as the motor habits and spirit of the past of the race, persisting in the present, as rudimentary organs."[14]

and again:

"Thus the boy is father of the man in a new sense, in that his qualities are infinitely older, and existed, well compacted, untold ages before the more distinctly human attributes were developed."

Hall, at the same time, places overwhelming emphasis upon muscular development.

"Muscles", he writes, "are in a most intimate and peculiar sense the organs of the will. They have built all the roads, cities, and machines in the world, written all the books, spoken all the words, and, in fact, done everything that man has accomplished with matter. Character might be in a sense defined as a plexus of motor habits."

Sully, as a psychologist, viewed play objectively and with less moral bias than Froebel or Stanley Hall, but unlike Groos and Hall, he did not attach a specialised function to play. Indeed, he cast doubts on the assumption that the adult, with his superior understanding, would easily comprehend this activity of his intellectual inferiors. In his *Studies of Childhood*[15] he says, talking of children at play:

"We talk . . . glibly about their play, their make-believe, their illusions; but how much do we really know of their state of mind when they act out a little scene of domestic life or of the battlefield?"

To Sully, children's play was essentially the expression of childish imagination and ideas. There was imitative play on the one hand, which copied those adult activities constantly seen, and there was play that expressed ideas conjured up by a vivid imagination fed by stories from books and by things seen and not completely understood.

Later, for example, in the chapter from which the above quotation is taken, he says of play:

"The source of play is the impulse to realise a bright idea: whence, as we shall see by and by, its close kinship to art as a whole."

Sully conceives play as essentially the spontaneous activity of the child. He lays particular stress upon the difficulty of observing children's play, and he gives more than one striking example of children distressed at adult interruption of their play—interruption either by physical interference or by failure to enter into the play then in progress. For example, in Chapter II he relates the following story told him by a mother:

" A little girl of four was playing shops with her younger sister. 'The elder one was shopman at the time I came into her room and kissed her. She broke out into piteous sobs, I could not understand why. At last she sobbed out: "Mother, you never kiss the man in the shop." I had with my kiss quite spoilt her illusion.'"

He nowhere essays a survey of the whole field of play.

If we would, therefore, attempt the task of passing the field of children's play in review, it is to Stanley Hall and to Groos that we must turn for classification of the forms of play and for theories of the meaning of play. There are, however, considerable difficulties in the way of acceptance of the views put forward by either.

To consider first the standpoint of Karl Groos:

The first difficulty that appears is that Groos nowhere separates the play of children from the play of adult men and women. He classifies as play many activities which, when practised by adults, are indeed play, but when performed by children, if ever this occurs, they have a different significance. (See, for example, the sections on Perception of Form, and on Memory and Recognition.[12])

Groos further makes no distinction between activities which are undertaken by a child in its normal process of gaining control of the muscles of its body, and play. For example, he writes:

" Almost as soon as the child has learned to preserve his equilibrium in ordinary walking, he proceeds to complicate the problem by trying to walk on curbstones, in a rut, on a beam, on a balustrade or narrow wall."

While Groos classes this as play, because in an adult it would be play, in a child it is not play, but serious effort at motor control. That is to say, activities of this kind are the parallel in childhood of the gradual undertaking of more and more difficult tasks that an adult sets himself in the enterprise of learning a difficult exercise, and are not in any sense play at all.

As a result, Groos fails to distinguish between movements made by the child in the effort to gain control over his body, which are to the child purely purposive in function, and movements and activities made by the child for the sake only of the pleasure they bring. The classification of group play into fighting plays, love plays, etc., makes Groos's work inapplicable to the activities of the ordinary child at play in a civilised country, as will be found by anyone who attempts to put these classifications into practice. Finally many important aspects of children's play are omitted altogether; for example, all infantile play, and all such play as is described in Chapter IV of this book.

Stanley Hall, on the other hand, takes play almost exclusively as motor play—indeed, states that "play is motor poetry." At one point in *Youth: Its Education, Regimen, and Hygiene*[14], he writes:

"The field of play is as wide as life and its varieties far outnumber those of industries and occupations in the census."

This promises well, but he goes on to say:

"Play and games differ in seasons, sex, and age. McGhee has shown, on the basis of some 8,000 children, that running plays are pretty constant for boys from six to seventeen but that girls are always far behind boys, and run steadily less from eight to eighteen. In games of choice, boys showed a slight rise at sixteen and seventeen, and girls a rapid increase at eleven and a still more rapid one after sixteen. In games of imitation girls excel and show a marked, as boys do a slight, pubescent fall. In those games involving rivalry boys at first greatly excel girls, but are overtaken by the latter in the eighteenth year, both showing marked increment. Girls have the largest number of plays and specialise on a few less than boys, and most of these plays are of the unorganised kinds."

This shows he has again only "games" in mind; a viewpoint which is shared by Helen Marshall, one of the most recent writers on *Children's Plays, Games, and Amusements*[7].

Finally, in this century, Professor Freud put forward a different view. In *Beyond the Pleasure Principle*[16] he analyses the play of a single child of eighteen months, and writes as follows:

"We see that children repeat in their play everything that has made a great impression on them in actual life, that they thereby abreact the strength of the impression and so to speak make themselves masters of the situation. But on the other hand it is clear enough that all their play is influenced by the dominant wish of their time of life: viz. to be grown-up and to be able to do what grown-up people do. It is also observable that the unpleasing character of the experience does not always prevent its being utilised as a game. . . In the play of children we seem to arrive at the conclusion that the child repeats even the unpleasant experiences because through his own activity he gains a far more thorough mastery of the strong impression than was possible by mere passive experience. Every fresh repetition seems to strengthen this mastery for which the child strives."

He also relates play to an impulse to repetition:

" In the light of such observations as these, drawn from the behaviour during transference and from the fate of human beings, we may venture to make the assumption that there really exists in psychic life a repetition-compulsion which goes beyond the pleasure-principle. We shall now also feel disposed to relate to this compelling force the dreams of shock-patients and the play-impulse in children."

This conception of play has been developed by the psycho-analytic school into a theory by which play is regarded exclusively as the representation in symbolic form of wishes, ideas, and thoughts related to the theory of infantile sexuality. This view of play, primarily put forward by Melanie Klein, has been further developed by M. N. Searl and Dr. M. Schmideberg. For further exposition of this conception reference can be made to papers by these authors published in the *International Journal of Psycho-Analysis.**

While it will be perfectly clear from many of the extracts which follow, that play of the kind described by the psycho-analytic school does certainly exist, it is the contention of the present writer that just as the views put forward by Groos and Hall do not cover the whole range of children's play, this conception also cannot be taken to cover more than a certain part of the total field of children's play.

There is, therefore, at present no theory of play available which can be applied to all forms taken by the play of children, and, further, there exists as yet no comprehensive survey of these forms from an analysis of which such a theory could be constructed. It is the purpose of the present volume to attempt to lay down the ground plan for such a survey.

In the view of the writer, play in children is the expression of the child's relation to the whole of life, and no theory of play is possible which is not also a theory which will cover the whole of a child's relation to life. Play in the sense, therefore, in which it will be used in this book, is taken as applying to all activities in children that are spontaneous and self-generated; that are ends in themselves; and that are unrelated to "lessons" or to the normal physiological needs of the child's own day.

The question of the nature of a suitable classification under which all types of play can be presented is a problem which, although vitally important, is too large for discussion at this point. Reasons, however, for the form of classification adopted and the principles upon which it is based will be found in Chapter XI.

---

*See Bibliography at the end of the Introduction.

CHAPTER II

THE OBSERVATION OF PLAY

"A child is very quick in spying whether he is being observed, and as soon as he suspects you are especially interested in his talk, he is apt to try to produce an effect."

JAMES SULLY.

THE PRESSING PROBLEM which next arises is: what kind of children can be selected for observation, and in what manner can they be observed? Susan Isaacs, in the Introduction to her study on *Intellectual Growth in Young Children*[17], puts succinctly the difficulty of observation and of presentation of the facts observed:

"The selection of instances to illustrate or demonstrate a particular psychological generalisation . . . commonly means that the reader sees the material on which the generalisation is based, only at the remove of the writer's judgment. The act of selection is itself an act of judgment. . . It may be . . . that contrary instances are overlooked, or their importance minimised; it may be . . . that the general context of any piece of behaviour might, if given, put a different colour upon things . . ."

Such selection is the basis of laboratory work, and, although inevitable, it carries with it certain dangers.

"By looking for particular answers to particular questions," writes Susan Isaacs, "we run the risk of missing other perhaps more significant facts which might transform our problem and make our previous questions idle. The interrelations of our different attempts to find the connecting threads between the partial reports of the experimental method often disclose new and more fundamental problems. The last word has to come from the survey of larger wholes."

The present book is no freer than any other work from these difficulties. An endeavour has been made to meet them by an attempt to bring together observations from as many sources as possible demonstrating as wide a variety of forms of children's play as could be collected. Such selection as has been made is concerned only with the grouping of these observations. It is unlikely that this collection of material is exhaustive, and no claim is made by the author for completeness; all that can be said is that the best possible effort has been made to omit no crucial evidence.

As regards the presentation of the material: in every case where practicable the actual words of the observer have been given, and the quotations placed as nearly as possible in relation to their context. The sex and age of the children mentioned are given with each selection, and by comparison of initials the different play forms of individual children may be traced. The choice of cases out of which the extracts have been taken has been quite arbitrary, and follows no rules, the bulk of the case material available making an exhaustive review of it both impossible and unsuitable.

The next point that arises is, how is the play of children to be observed without disturbing the play itself, and how are the observations to be recorded?

Children are only entirely spontaneous in play when they are alone and undisturbed by adult comment. Very young children, it is true, are largely unaware of unobtrusive adult observation, and with them the difficulty is lessened. It is also true that rare adults at times succeed in being, when with children, so unobtrusively engaged upon their own work that the children grow really to be unaware of their presence. Yet it is uncommon for such people to pay close attention to what is going on around them, or to make records of the play they see.

In an interesting discussion of this problem, Mrs. Isaacs[17] points out the distorting factor that is introduced, for example, into Stern's exhaustive observation of his own children[18] by the operation of parental standards of behaviour.

"An examination of some of the contributions of genetic psychologists", she writes, "makes it clear that a very great number of supposed psychological observations are permeated through and through by pedagogic influences and moral judgments, and that the psychologists in question are themselves quite unaware of this, and therefore unable to make any allowance for it in their own conclusions. . .

"If this view be soundly based, it is obviously one of the utmost importance for child psychologists. It means that we can never entirely rule ourselves out as a factor, even should we approximate to the pure observer, and interfere as little as possible with the children we are watching. But where we actually combine the two functions of educator and observer, and, above all, when we are the actual *parents* of the children in question, as well as psychologists, many allowances will have to be made in all our records for our own direct if involuntary effect upon the children's behaviour."

An even more drastic example of the same phenomenon is supplied by Sully, who, in a study of children's lies, says:

" To begin with those little ruses and dissimulations which, according to M. Perez, are apt to appear almost from the cradle in the case of certain children, it is plainly difficult to bring them into the category of full-fledged lies. When, for example, a child wishing to keep a thing hides it, and on your asking for it holds out empty hands, it would be hard to name this action a lie, even though there is in it a germ of deception. . . Anybody who has observed children's play and dramatic talk, and knows how readily and completely they can imagine the non-existent so as to lose sight of the existent, will be chary, when talking of them, of using the word lie. There may be solemn sticklers for truth who would be shocked to hear the child when at play saying, ' I am a coachman ', ' Dolly is crying ', and so forth. But the discerning see nothing to be alarmed at here."

This influence of the factor of parental standards can be traced throughout the work of the older observers.

The obstacle presented to the free play of children by the presence of an adult is, therefore, not the size of the adult, though this does also play a rôle, but his standards. The scale of values of an adult is so radically different from the scale of values of a child, his prohibitions and permissions differ so fundamentally from those natural to a child, as also do his interests and his impulses, that there can be no common ground between adult *qua* adult and child, and no means by which the watching adult is not felt by the child as the criticising adult.

The *impasse*, therefore, facing the enterprise of impersonal observation of play appears complete.

The real nature of this difficulty is to be found in the last quotation from Mrs. Isaacs. If the watching adult stands in the relation of observer, educator, or parent, there is no solution of the problem but that which she suggests. But it is the thesis of the work upon which this book is based that circumstances can be created in which these difficulties can be very largely eliminated, and the play of children seen without material distortion. That is to say, that there is a rôle which an adult can fill when with children, which does not come within the description of observer, educator, or parent. A situation can be created between adult and child where the adult characteristics that make him a judge in the eyes of the child are very greatly modified, and where for all intents and purposes, from the child's point of view, the adult ceases to be an adult and becomes a comrade instead.

It is not possible here to give a description of the technique employed in creating this situation, as too many issues are involved, but some conception of the method may be gathered from comparison of the extracts that form the bulk of this book with similar records made by other observers. It is the fact that the purpose of the Institute is not the education but the study and the curative treatment of the children it observes that gives it its unique opportunity for the study of children at play.

In order that the records later quoted can be understood, a very brief description of the work of the Institute must be given here.

The Institute of Child Psychology is an out-patient institution designed for the treatment and study of children. These children come actually from all classes of society, but the main bulk from the elementary schools. They fall into the four following classes:

1. Children suffering from disturbances of their emotional life: anxiety, night terrors, fears, inhibitions, nervousness, etc.

2. Children suffering from chronic disorders, such as epilepsy, asthma, catarrh, debility, constipation, enuresis.

3. Children who are unable to adjust themselves socially:

(a) At home, e.g. quarrelling, jealousy, excessive timidity, inability to bear separation from parents.

(b) At school, e.g. bullying, sneaking, unmanageableness, truancy.

(c) Generally, e.g. stealing, lying, hooliganism, destructiveness.

4. Children with educational difficulties, e.g. failure in concentration, inability to learn particular subjects, mirror-writing, word-blindness.

An intelligence test is given by a worker with whom the child is unfamiliar, to every child before its entry to the playroom. Mentally deficient children are excluded.

Children are accepted at the Institute at any age from one to eighteen years. These children visit the Institute twice weekly only for two and a half hours at a time. They are none of them resident. For the most part parents bring the children, but they spend the time in a separate room, and *are not on any account admitted to the playroom* (a very occasional exception to this rule is made in the case of very shy children on their first visit).

As the Institute is both a training and a research body, an endeavour is made so to group children in the playroom that no age and no sex shall predominate, and that the type of temperament and of difficulty presented by the children shall cover as wide a field as possible.

NOTES ON THE TECHNIQUE OF OBSERVATION EMPLOYED

As has been explained already, the Institute, being not only an out-patient institution for the treatment of children, but a centre for psychological observation and training, has set itself to evolve a technique of the handling and observation of children which will overcome the difficulties we have described. This method of observation is based upon the following principles:

The Institute accepts the fact that observations cannot satisfactorily be made without the actual presence of an adult among the children.

Since from a child's point of view the disadvantage of an adult as a companion in play is not his size but his standards and tastes, adults working in the playroom are submitted to a form of training directed towards enabling them, when in contact with the children, to accept the children's point of view as far as possible as their own.

In doing so the following general rules are continuously allowed:

Rule 1. As regards size. In normal contact with an adult, the child is always conscious of his own small stature. In the playroom this is minimised by the adult placing himself on the child's level or below it.

Rule 2. As concerns the relation of the child to the worker.

(*a*) Workers in the playroom are considered by children and staff as the friends of the children, but at the same time the usual rôle of child and adult is reversed. Every adult in the playroom is absolutely at the disposal of the child or children with whom he or she is playing, and carries out without question the orders of the children, except where these would result in damage or danger to the child.

(*b*) The standards of behaviour in the playroom are the standards of children and not of adults.

(*c*) In *no* case does the adult allow himself to be enticed by the child into administering blame, and in no case is reproof to be administered by an adult; awkward situations must be evaded rather than directly opposed.

(*d*) No spontaneous adverse comment is made by the worker on the children's use of the toys and materials, however apparently mis-directed. Every action of every child is accepted as obvious and right, without reference to the question of the appropriate or inappropriate use of the materials to hand, unless there is another piece of apparatus in the playroom which would carry out the desired aim more effectively, in which case the worker would draw the child's attention to it.

The children are allowed to move as freely as they like from occupation to occupation, and only rarely is an attempt made to induce them to persevere at any one occupation. (It should be clearly understood that these rules apply *only* to behaviour within the playroom.)

Every child during his hours in the Institute spends some time at rhythm and music.

PLAY MATERIAL AND THE CIRCUMSTANCES OF PLAY

Children playing freely out of doors, with space in which to roam and an adequate number of tools at hand, secure for themselves the material they need for their play. Children indoors are, on the contrary, entirely dependent upon the materials provided by grown-ups for their use.

It was Froebel[19] who first realised the existence of an intimate essential relationship between the material available for a child to handle and the development of the child's mind and emotions.

"To realise his aims," he wrote, "man, and more particularly the child, requires material, though it be only a bit of wood or a pebble with which he makes something or which he makes into something";

"The purpose of playthings and occupation material in general, is to aid the child freely to express what lies within him—to bring the phenomena of the outer world nearer to him, and thus to serve as mediator between the mind and the world."

Froebel arrived at his point of view by intuitive sympathy with the children under his care, but the same point has recently been made from another angle by Dr. Charlotte Bühler in her study of the effect of material upon the general maturation of children.[20] Summing up her conclusions, she writes:

"And now, finally, the question: What consequence and effect does the activity with material really have on the development of the child, and indeed on the development of mankind..? The absence of practical activity, the lack of experience in all practical things of life, seems, therefore, one of the important factors in determining the whole level of development of the child."

The question of the relation of the material used to the phantasy in the mind of the child will be found discussed in Chapter V of this book.

At the time of the founding of the I.C.P. (then the Children's Clinic) no examination had been made, as far as the writer has been able to ascertain, of the type of materials spontaneously chosen by children in play. It was our first task, therefore, to work out a selection of equipment which would supply the child with such materials as he would himself be able to discover in natural, i.e. country, surroundings.

The equipment now in use at the Institute has been selected partly through the observation of children at play in natural conditions, and partly by a process of trial and error in suiting this material to actual children's needs at the I.C.P.

In this way there has been built up a range of standardised material which is in constant use, and it has been a matter of very great interest to all at work in the Institute to find on the publication of Professor Bühler's paper in 1933 the high degree of comparability between the material freely selected by her children and that designed for use at the Institute.

The material available for the children's use at the Institute may be classified as follows:

PHANTASY MATERIAL. (Inchoate)* i.e. Material for the expression of phantasy.	Water and water toys, earth, sand, dough, modelling materials, paper-cutting materials, wood shapes and blocks, rods and holes.
(Choate)	"Worlds", mosaics, trains, "grotesques", materials for free drawing and painting, and for acting.
CONSTRUCTION MATERIAL.	Model-making, as Meccano, Kliptiko, etc. Paper pasting and cutting, sewing, weaving, etc. Carpentry and chemical toys.
HOUSE OR MINIATURE ADULT MATERIAL.	Dolls, house, shop, brooms, cooking utensils, etc., mincing machine and grinder.
MATERIALS GIVING SCOPE FOR MOVEMENT AND DESTRUCTION.	(Grinding and mincing.) Cutting and piercing instruments, skittles, rubber balls, and darts.

PHANTASY MATERIAL
INCHOATE

WATER AND WATER TOYS

All this material is placed near a sink, which is fitted with accessible taps and rubber tubing for attaching to the taps. The sink is shallow enough for little children to be able to pull out the plug themselves, and deep enough to sail boats in. A movable high wooden step makes it accessible to quite small children.

Most easily procurable of the water toys are rubber, celluloid, wood, and tin toys that can sink and float. Then come toy baths, bathrooms, and lavatories with working parts, kettles, teapots, cans from which water can be poured, soap-bubble pipes, water pistols, and boats.

*Explanation of these terms will occur in later chapters.

EARTH AND SAND

Inchoate mouldable material is supplied by *Sand* in white, light brown, and dark brown varieties that make intriguing colour differences and serve to express different forms of phantasy. For example, the brown can represent earth; the white, snow; the mixed brown and white seashore, etc.

Earth is not used in the playroom, and its use is reserved for gardening experiments in the garden, but if desired, it can be very well used in a tray.

Sand and *Sand and Water* lend themselves to the demonstration of a large variety of phantasies, as, for example, tunnel-making, burying or drowning, land and seascapes. When wet, the sand may be moulded, and when dry it is pleasant to feel, and many tactile experiments can be made with the gradual addition of moisture. Wet sand can be dried up again and reconverted to wet, or by adding further water it becomes " slosh ", and finally water when the dry land has completely disappeared.

Sand is used in a waterproof tray 18 in. by 27 in., with a rim 1¾ in. deep, made of wood and zinc lined.

Dough and Clay. Closely allied to water and sand are a number of other substances, but there are dangers connected with their use. Sand is familiar to children, and familiarity has dulled the edge of stimulation, but other substances are new, and, for reasons that lie in the deeper regions of the psyche, they are powerfully stimulating to infantile emotion. The chief of these intermediate substances are *Modeller's Clay* and *Flour*.

Children, when handling these materials at school or at home, are under supervision, and are struggling with a somewhat refractory material; they are trying to make something, or are imitating an adult in trying to cook. The child's attention is therefore held by the thing he is trying to make and by learning how to do it. In struggling to obey the directions he is given, and to master the material itself, the child's whole being is absorbed, and the emotional dangers that so readily arise in the use of this material are avoided. In the laboratory playroom of the Institute this idea of an ultimate use for the material is absent. The material is there for the children to experiment with, and no restrictions are put on the manner of its use. The dangers in the use of this material, to which reference has been made, lie in its likeness to certain very primitive interests of the human being, interests which in the process of civilising the individual come early under ban. Experiment, therefore, in a permissive atmosphere with this material involves certain definite risks to the whole structure that the mind has built up against the direct realisation of very primitive desires. These desires and their influence upon play will be considered in Chapter IV. This material should exist in the equipment of every children's psychological surgery, but only for use with observers perfectly aware of the dangers inherent in it, and who have adequate training and experience.

MODELLING MATERIALS

After dough and clay come two substances whose consistency cannot be greatly varied, and are, therefore, without the dangers attendant on flour and dough. These are *Plasticine Substances* and *Coloured Wax*. *Plasticine Substances* form an invaluable part of any apparatus for psychological work with children and can be used in a large number of ways. The substance is essentially mouldable, and can be satisfactorily cut and chopped. *Coloured Wax* is not so mouldable and cuts poorly. It is, however, bright and clear in colour and sets hard, and can be pulled into very fine lengths. The purpose served by the two substances is quite different, and the playroom is, therefore, stocked with both.

SOLID OBJECTS FOR PHANTASY EXPRESSION

Wood Shapes and Blocks. All these are of non-splintering wood. They are of infinite variety in size, shape, and colour, and are used to depict a very wide range of scenes and imaginative phantasies. Instances of the use of these bricks will be found in Chapter V, and of the use of rods and holes in Chapter IV.

Coloured Paper Shapes. Coloured paper, both gummed and plain, already cut into shapes or in sheets, for use in ways with which Čizek has made us familiar, serves many purposes. To it should be added plain white paper and scissors.

CHOATE MATERIALS

" *The World.*" Every child forms conceptions of the outside world at a very early age. Part of the work of the playroom laboratory is to provide material by which these concepts can be demonstrated and manipulated so that inter-relations between them may become manifest. In what is known as the "world" cabinet of the playroom the child can find material for the expression of these ideas. The cabinet consists of a series of trays upon which cheap miniature models of practically every ordinary object are arranged in classes easily grasped by the child. This "world" cabinet is in general used in connection with a sand tray, and placed beside it at a point that makes all objects readily accessible to the child.

Painting and Drawing Materials. These serve the purposes both of choate and inchoate phantasy. They include crayons, chalks, pencils, brushes, rags, and two kinds of paints—powder paints and moist colour blocks, and "grotesques" of various kinds (see p. 191).

CONSTRUCTION

Material. Many of the commercially produced constructive toys, Meccano, Kliptiko, etc., and many simple forms of motor-car and house construction come in usefully here. In addition, there should be a carpenter's bench and carpentry tools. For girls a collection of handcraft material, such as weaving, fancy-work, basket-work, etc., is valuable. These give outlet for constructive energies, fill gaps when phantasy work has been too stimulating, and offer possibilities of reassurance to timid children convinced of their incapacity for any form of achievement.

HOUSE MATERIALS

Shop, Dolls, Prams, and Household Utensils. These give children instruments with which to dramatise the everyday life they share in and see happening around them. Toy brooms, brushes, etc., are often included in the ordinary toys given to children; the only way in which those used at the Institute differ is that they must be really serviceable and workable, and only toy-like in that they are smaller editions of the real thing. These toys are not merely used by the children for imitating the often incomprehensible actions of the adult world they see around them, but they furnish instruments with which the children can dramatise their versions of everyday life, and their conceptions of how they would *like* life to be. Studies of the use of this material will be found in Chapter VI.

MOVEMENT AND DESTRUCTION

Opportunities for movement can easily be supplied in many ways by ball games, rhythm work, and running games, but provision for the expression of destructive impulses requires more consideration.

Destruction. The desire to destroy, since it is so rigorously suppressed by adult society, must be given special opportunities for satisfaction in the playroom, if the impulse is to be really accessible for study; and, moreover, if it is to be "played through" in such a way as to clear the road for constructive effort. Three types of destructive action are provided for: skittles, where the objects are merely knocked down and rolled over, hammer toys, grinding and mincing, where the chestnuts, etc., are put into a grinder and reduced to powder; and throwing and cutting-up games with plasticine. Many of the constructive implements such as are used in leather-work, punching, etc., can also be employed as outlets for destructive energy.

TRAINS, ETC.

Trains fill many gaps in play and are used for many purposes and for children of all ages.

There are are also *Pull-along Toys* for little children.

RHYTHM AND MUSIC

The rhythm room needs to be considered separately, and for the notes that follow, and for those in Chapter III, I am indebted to Miss M. Kirschner, rhythm mistress at the Institute. She writes:

"The apparatus of the rhythm room is as simple as possible. There is plenty of space, a clean floor, something soft for the children to lie on, and there are also a few clothes from the acting cupboard and a number of balls. The actual musical instruments include drums, tambourines, bells, two or three mouth-organs, tin whistles, and a gramophone and a piano.

"The children may, therefore, *move freely*, and *play* and *listen*, and can combine music and movement.

"What use do the children make of this?

"It must be remembered that in the rhythm room the initiative is left to the children as far as possible, in exactly the same way as is done in the playroom. Working with rhythm and music, we are in the same favourable position as are workers in the playroom, in that musical instruments call forth a natural response in the children in the same way that is observed with the play material. Not only does the general aspect of an instrument invite the child to play it, but different types of instrument call out different types of use. On the percussion instruments children will experiment with rhythm, tone, and musical form; on the simple melodic instruments they gain their first experience of the pitch of sound and melody; while on the piano there is the combination of melody, sound, and harmony.

"While the instruments themselves invite the children to make use of them, there is no such direct invitation for them to use their bodies. They are, as it were, used to their bodies. The manner in which they use them depends largely upon the training they have had in games, drill, and dancing at school, and upon the surroundings in which they have been brought up. Some children are induced by sight of the clear floor space to repeat exercises they have already learned; with others, music will give the necessary spark to entice them to activity, and they will dance spontaneously. If, however, they do not respond spontaneously to the natural stimulus the room provides, a stimulus is given by suggesting the idea of a circus, where they become "performers" and do acrobatics, or the idea of a zoo, in which they imitate animals, and call upon the worker to guess what animals they represent. In every case what is aimed at is the free expression of the child's response to sound, rhythm, melody, and movement, and the development of his capacity to create these for himself. *In no case are already composed pieces of music or dancing taught to the children.*"

RECORDS

It now remains to consider in what manner records can be made of play carried out by the children in the play and rhythm rooms.

From the scientific standpoint, the value of any observation depends upon the accuracy with which it is reported. The problem of accurately recording work of this kind is a particularly difficult one. If the children are to feel themselves free, no notes may be taken in their presence. In the playroom the children move, produce, and destroy scenes, create games, and speak, and no literal account of any of these activities can be given. Experiment has often shown the unreliability of witnesses, even in favourable circumstances.[21] Although there are steps which can be taken to guard against this element of fallacy, certain fallacies have to be accepted as inherent in the reporting of all observations. An absolutely accurate record of children's play, accurate in the sense that barometric readings are accurate, cannot in the nature of things be made. It must therefore be accepted that certain types of error inevitably creep in, and that there are errors which arise from the essential structure of the observer's mind. Such types of error, for example, are the following:

1. The mind cannot grasp that which is wholly unfamiliar to it. No matter how often the evidence for a fact be repeated, if there is no knowledge already in the mind to which this experience can be linked the new fact will remain unperceived.

2. The mind is more apt to see that which it has already noticed. The working of this principle is usefully shown when a child is moved from a familiar worker to a new one. It is true that often a fresh worker induces, almost in spite of him or herself, a change of play, but it is also true, and very important, that often when play has been similar and the observer new, when the account is written up, the emphasis proves to be differently distributed, and new features are brought to light. These have been present all along, but have not been previously reported.

3. The mind is unable to see that which it has not been trained to accept. The work of Freud, and indeed of the whole of the analytical or dynamic school of thought, displays this rule. The facts of human nature and of the sexual development of the human being were the same in the days of Pharoah as now, and they required no special instrument for observation, but, owing to mankind's unwillingness to accept what it saw, these facts remained unnoticed until the end of the last century.

4. The mind unconsciously distorts what it hears and sees, according to its own prejudices. This is not the same fallacy as is noted in types 2 and 3, where facts are omitted altogether from the mind's record of events. It is the process by which the facts seen and recorded are so distorted in the record that the meaning conveyed to the reader is often out of all harmony with the facts as they originally occurred. This form of inaccuracy happens when strong emotions are aroused in the observer, which render a particular distortion of an event more pleasurable to the individual than the actual occurrence. The pages of any political controversy will supply abundant examples of this rule.

That mental mechanisms of this kind become active in the apparently detached or impersonal work of watching a roomful of children at play, as also the direction in which these mechanisms are likely to work, are shown in the quotations from Sully given above. Early personal difficulties, for example, with aggression, with curiosity, and with spitefulness, make these qualities very difficult to tolerate in other people, and therefore very hard to recognise in the children with whom we play. Moreover, an adult is apt to project on to children ideas he has already formed of childhood, and to see children, not as they are, but as he wishes them to be.

For all these reasons accurate observation of children at play is an undertaking the difficulty of which should not be under-estimated, and for the present, and until our knowledge has very widely increased, all records of the moods and play of children need, before acceptance, to be given careful and intensive scrutiny.

To minimise the operation of fallacies in making records, certain precautions are continuously taken in the Institute. They are as follows:

1. For every session in the playroom a time-sheet is kept. On it is recorded in sequence the activities of each child during its time in the playroom, and the names of the worker or workers with whom he has played. This book is in full view of the children, and is an event of such steady routine that so far no child has shown any emotional disturbance in regard to it. The older children sometimes help to fill it in. When secretarial time allows, a personal record is made monthly from this book and on this sheet the child's disposition of time is recorded, with the names of workers who have played with him, and the apparatus that has been used.

2. Immediately after each play session, each worker writes an account of the play of the child with whom he or she has played.

3. The technique of reporting is carefully taught to workers in the playroom, and discussed at seminars, and special coaching is given to those who find making or reporting observations difficult.

4. All reports are collected together on the day prior to the next session and by assembled workers compared with each other and with the time-book; discrepancies are then investigated and made good.

5. Friendly discussion and comparison amongst workers tend to bring to light characteristic individual difficulties in observation, and so to check reports. For example, a curious phenomenon reported successively in several children by the same worker is likely to have a subjective origin, while the same fact reported in the same child by different observers has probably objective value.

6. Study of the imagery native to the worker reveals sources of inevitable

weakness in reporting, for which suitable exercises in attention can slowly compensate; for example, some workers can only remember things heard, some only things seen, and so on.

7. Comparison of report with report and correlation of reports over a wide period bring to light definite trends that can be used later as further checks on fresh reports.

8. Change of child from worker to worker, the use of a more practised worker to check the work of a less skilled observer, all help, if sufficient allowance be made for the effect of the personality of the worker on the child, to obtain reliability.

9. Finally, some personal analysis of the worker by the method of any recognised school is a potent aid to observation. Since each school lays emphasis upon a particular type of fact, as well as opening his eyes to his own unconscious motivation in his reactions to the children, it trains the worker to look for this order of fact in the children. But even here it is wise for the group of workers to include amongst themselves those who have had personal experience of *several different* schools of thought, since it is inevitable that a human mind acclaims as truth that which it has itself successfully experienced, and, recognising others as akin to itself, feels that this truth is absolute and all other error or illusion. It is valuable, therefore, to have the children regarded at one and the same time from several points of view.

10. To illustrate the work, where possible, all children's drawings, etc., are kept and filed in the case-sheet. In the case of " worlds ", before they are destroyed, diagrams are made and filed appropriately in the case-sheets.

All work, such as plays, stories, etc., done by the children and brought to the Institute, is kept and duly filed in the case-sheet. Each case-sheet is sub-divided so that workers' reports and children's work are filed in separate positions.

Finally, all the conclusions put forward in the following chapters have first been submitted for discussion to the audience to whom the original lectures were delivered.

SOURCES OF RECORD

The sources from which the notes given in this book are taken are the records of 229 children who have attended the Institute between the years October 1928 and July 1934. The figure overleaf gives the age distribution of these children on entry.

For 144 of these children complete records were available, covering all sides of the children's lives, home circumstances and heredity, physical

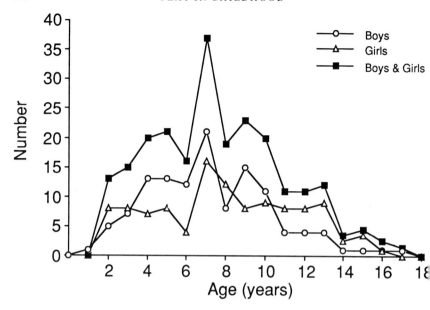

history and present conditions, intelligence tests, school reports, and family evaluations, together with full reports of all play carried out in the Institute playroom laboratory. The periods of attendance of these children varied from four to a hundred and eighty attendances.

The Intelligence Quotients of these children varied from 65 to 141 and the larger number fell betwen 85 and 115. For very young children no estimate of intelligence was attempted owing to the absence of really reliable tests for these ages. In certain cases attendance at the Institute materially altered the level of intellectual quotient; a girl of six, for example, entering the Institute in May 1933, when tested in June 1933 gave an I.Q. of 82, with a base line of 4. On discharge in September 1934 she was re-tested by the same observer, and gave at this date an I.Q. of 111, with a base line of 7.

It is this consideration which modifies the statement made upon p. 27 that no mentally defective child is accepted. There has been devised for use at the Institute a Mosaic Test* which is given to all children on admission to the Institute and which is repeated at intervals during their attendance. This consists in the presentation to the subject of a number of carefully selected geometrical shapes in black, white, and four clear colours—red, blue, yellow, and green—for use in the making of a free design. No restriction is placed

---

*A volume on the standardisation of this test is now in the course of preparation. [*Editor's note*: Lowenfeld, M. (1954) *The Lowenfeld Mosaic Test*. London: Newman Neame.]

upon the number of pieces used or the time taken. After completion the
design is carefully copied and recorded. Children of from five upwards are
capable of carrying out this test. By study and comparison of large numbers
of designs so obtained correlations have been discovered which make these
designs a valuable aid in estimating emotional stability, and by means of
these designs it is becoming possible to distinguish between educational or
intellectual retardation due to emotional blocking and educational and
intellectual retardation which arise from inherent mental defect.

The age distribution of these 144 children on entry is given in the
following figure:

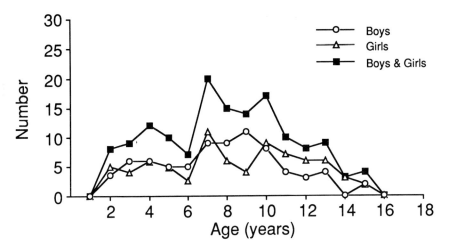

CHAPTER III

PLAY AS BODILY ACTIVITY

"It has been stated as a fundamental truth that the plays and occupations of children should by no means be treated as offering merely means for passing time, hence as mere outer activity, but rather that by means of such plays and employments the child's innermost nature must be satisfied."

FRIEDRICH FROEBEL.[19]

W E COME NOW to a discussion of the groups into which children's play can fall, and to an attempt to see the meaning these activities bear to the children who engage in them. We have agreed already that all play is active, and it is fitting that the first form of play to be observed in infants is that of bodily activity.

Play as Bodily Activity falls into six sub-groups:

1. What is called by Charlotte Bühler "Function Play".[22]
2. Purposeless and unco-ordinated movement (usually associated with noise), commonly described as "letting off steam".
3. Certain loose forms of physical play which express banned primitive impulses.
4. Rhythmic movements and the enjoyment of rhythm.
5. Forms of physical play which express certain very deep emotional states that are not commonly recognised in ordinary life.
6. Plays of personification; out of which grow drama.

Spencer[9] put forward a theory that the child is driven to play because he has more brain energy than he can use in any other way, and therefore works it off on play. As has been pointed out in Chapter I, there are many objections to this theory as offering a complete explanation of children's play. Nevertheless, careful study of children at play shows that there are a number of forms of play that do fit in with this description. As a matter of interest, it is the games of which the essential activity is running that have hitherto been given chief prominence in the studies that have been made of children's play (e.g. see Marshall[7]).

Those varieties of running games in which the form is definite, and which are played according to rules, are discussed in Chapter VIII. In this chapter we have to consider the types of play in which the primary sentiment is the child's feeling of movement, and to examine the use he makes of this impulse, and its relation to the expression of his emotions.

The first form of play to be considered is that of which Professor Bühler makes a detailed study in her work on the *First Year of Life* [23], and to which she has given the name *Funktionspiel*.

1. "*Funktionspiel*" is the amusement a child gets from trying out his capacity to move first his own body, and then other objects, and the fun he gets from repeating the movements he has already achieved. Dr. Bühler gives an interesting discussion of this form of play and its relation to other kinds of play, to work, and to creation in *Kindheit und Jugend* [26], and in the section on *Scherz* and *Komik* shows how fun and *Funktionspiel* are the games of tiny infants (see p. 182 of this book).

2. "*Letting off Steam.*" Every healthy infant finds itself highly charged with emotion and energy. This energy and emotion have two main channels of discharge: by acquisition of muscular activity, and the exploration of sense experience.

For the first few years a child has no skill in the manipulation of his senses, and the channels of enjoyment of sense experience and intellectual experiment, which are open to every adult, are not at his disposal as avenues for the discharge of energy. If, therefore, he is to save himself from fretfulness and misery, he is compelled to allow a great deal of his energy to express itself instead through muscular activity.

Froebel, very early in his observations, noted that "boys spring into physical activity as mere expressions of buoyancy of spirits", and this observation will be endorsed by anyone with experience of children as equally true of boys and girls.

Exercise of the body, of the voice, of the whole person in production of the maximum possible commotion is an absolute necessity at some time or other to every healthy child. Noise is necessary, movement is necessary, and to be healthy these must be allowed to be exactly what they are—shapeless explosions of an overplus of energy, providing vivid examples of Spencer's theory of play.

Muscular activity of this sort has no aim and no shape. It takes the form of violent running up and down, the tumbling of one child over another, waving of arms, shouting, and skipping. It is a valuable means of reducing a charge of energy to that point at which the degree of interior tension felt by the child is more proportioned to the possibilities of co-ordinated expression which lie within his reach. If properly exercised, the right to "let off steam", when the need is felt, results in renewed power of concentration, and the re-awakening of interest in accomplishment. (This has been particularly the experience of certain infant schools where periodic "letting off steam" in lesson times has been permitted.)

The following are extracts from notes of cases at the I.C.P. which illustrate this type of energy discharge:

R.S., Boy, aged 9¼. He ran into the rhythm room and round the screen, on to the sofa, where he stood on his head, then he bounced up and down, sitting. He then rushed to the gramophone and shouted through the trumpet as another boy had done. He wanted " one more go ", and then another and another.

On another occasion. He was wildly exuberant, and dashed about while playing at skittles as if he could not keep still—up the stairs, on the lavatory roof, down the stairs, balancing on the outside of the banisters, etc., several times.

G.W., Girl, aged 13½. She threw and kicked the ball, saying spontaneously that she was letting off steam, and perhaps that was why she was also so fond of ball games. She said, " I love throwing the ball *at* something."

J.M., Boy, aged 10½. Rather out of hand playing with another boy. They were having a rough and tumble on the floor, singing " All Together ", and J.M. kicking A.B. At first he refused all suggestions of work, but later volunteered that he would like aeroplane construction. He began on this, but his attention was never caught. He called frequently to A.B., and to another boy, and made efforts to upset smaller children's work. Several times he ran over to snatch handfuls of wet sand and threatened to throw it. He dropped it on the floor and seemed to enjoy the feel of it. He then ran to A.B. and another boy and began a fresh rough and tumble.

Now it should be noted that to the small child the experience of muscle movement has two elements:

(*a*) The excitement of *discovery* of the self, of the outside world, and of growing power over both.

(*b*) The sheer joy of muscle movement (called by the psycho-analytic school " muscle erotism "), which finds its source in the pleasure experienced in the discharge of energy through muscular movement. This can first be seen in the movements of the whole body of an infant while suckling, and shows well in the vigorous movements of the arms and legs of a six months' old baby, playing on its back after its bath by the nursery fire.

Violent movement has the feeling tone to the individual who creates it, at any age, of being brilliant, loud-coloured, and noisy, and is accompanied in small children and in crowds by a strong desire for actual noise. The desire in children is expressed by whistling, shouting, and the banging of drums, and at an older age often develops into an intense pleasure in loud singing in chorus. Noise is inchoate, it has no shape, and is thus akin to the pressure of emotion within the child which itself also has as yet no shape. Further, noise is external, objective, a something produced *by* the child which everybody can hear, and therefore a comfort as a reassurance against the queerness and terror of the nameless, shapeless emotions within him. The noise, and the pleasure in noise, of the adolescent with a motor-bicycle is very much akin to this form of play.

For examples, entries regarding a boy of nine state:

A.T., Boy, aged 9. He grew more freely uproarious and finally took to tossing clouds of sand in the air with soldiers, guns, and all. He delighted in the power and chaos, and was very flushed at this point.

And concerning a group:

J.B., Boy aged 4, and F.V., Girl, aged 7. J.B. started playing with Matador. He got very excited, having made a pair of wheels, and he rolled them about the floor. His shouting attracted F.V., who joined him and made another pair of wheels. She was in a very excited mood, also shouting. She snatched a lot and threw her legs about. They both made what they called aeroplanes of very slight construction, chiefly for the purpose of dashing about with them, shouting and squirming on the floor.

Or a girl of 13:

M.E., Girl, aged 13. She was being most tiresome and very noisy, singing suddenly in an affected, music-hall voice music-hall songs, calling across the room, and generally interrupting everybody's work.

3. *The Expression in Group Play of Primitive Anti-social Impulses.* An angry child wandering disconsolately along a road will kick along a stone with satisfaction and relief to its feelings; it will arm itself with a stick taken from the hedge and use it to propel the stone, or an implement of power, waving and brandishing it in the air. Great is the satisfacton to be gained in so doing. The kicks are partly exercise of bodily movement, and belong therefore to the first group of active play, but they also give vent to feelings of exasperation and rage, spite and cruelty, just as an angered man, unable to give vent to his annoyance on the person who has provoked him, will relieve his feelings by chopping wood, or doing some other physically active work. For example, if a man actively at work on some physical task such as carpentering is called off to an errand which irritates him, when he goes back to work he will hammer or saw with an excessive abundance of "vicious" energy, and the work in consequence suffers rather than is benefited.

For a small child, outward expression of exasperation leads only to shame and punishment, and thus to further exasperation. Reproved by his elders, a small boy cannot retaliate, but will kick the table while he listens to the lecture. Some, at least, of the drive behind the imitation of national games, cricket and football, in city streets lies in the outlet given by them to primitive impulse of this kind.

Here are some I.C.P. notes in illustration:

K.W., Boy, aged 11. After some time, having achieved nothing, he joined another boy who was playing "football"—it was not suggested to him: he just drifted into the game after looking rather wistfully at it. He got very much the worst of it, as the other showed much more skill and he hardly touched the ball, nor did he make much effort to compete. Twice he was knocked over pretty hard, but he did not protest; he was his silent, withdrawn self, quietly taking the game as it came. But once, with a sudden spurt of what looked very much like fury, he kicked out with tremendous spirit. After this he subsided again, and the game ended when the other boy was too hot to go on. K.W. went on kicking the ball by himself, "shooting" between curtains at the door used as goal-posts.

A.T., Boy, aged 9. He was making a feint of hitting a girl with a hammer when he suddenly saw a lump of plasticine, and quickly rolled a bit into a small ball and hurled it at a worker who was at the other side of the room. This he repeated five or six times rapidly in succession. Another boy at this point wanted to join in, but the end of the playroom session ended what promised to be a battle royal. He was prepared to retaliate when the other became aggressive, but his own missiles were directed only against adults.

G.W., Girl, aged 13. She looked about the room and said she did not care for plasticine, but made a tortoise. She then said she would like to kick something to let off her feelings.

Play of this kind can occur in company or singly, but many children, to make it really effective, desire the approval of an audience.

Skittles and plasticine are used at the I.C.P. to explore this state of mind. The skittles are made in the shape of people, and often two children compete against each other. For example, some notes run:

B.R., Girl, aged 10. She had great satisfaction in knocking down a large number of skittles. In order to facilitate this, she suggested arranging the skittles close together. When another child joined the game and began to get the central interest, she showed discomfort and abreacted some of this violently in her next turn at the skittles.

A.T., Boy, aged 12. He placed the skittles close to each other, and refused worker's proposal that skilled players placed them apart. He demolished them five times, throwing the ball with tremendous force.*

B.G., Boy, aged 10. When playing with skittles with faces, he called one skittle his "Dad", another "Mum", others "Grandma" and "Grandad". He tried to hit "Grandad", or said he wanted to. Actually he put "Dad" immediately in front, so that it was difficult to hit "Grandad". Worker drew his attention to the fact that "Dad" was getting all the knocks, and he said, "That's not Dad." Then he said that the "Mum" skittle was "Dad". He played fairly, not minding when worker won. During the first part of the play he said, "I am a baby." Then he got into the wheel-chair and made worker wheel him up and down.

L.C., Girl, aged 10. One skittle was called by the child "Duffer" and made to stand in front of the others. She says "Duffer" is a boy, and "he is turning round to the others because he's tired of being out there alone." Then she put him back with the others.

B.C., Girl, aged 11½. She readily accepted the idea of playing skittles with G.W. (Girl). She aimed very accurately and knocked them all down nearly every time. Some of the skittles were called "Mother", "Father", "Brother", "Uncle".

The same kind of use of the resemblance shown by dolls to particular human beings for the explosion of negative emotions has been reported by Stanley Hall.[13]

"F. I had one doll which I never liked, because it resembled a very disagreeable person. We used to hang this doll on the clothes-line and take turns throwing stones at it."

A curious and interesting fact which has been occasionally observed with these children, and for which at the moment we have in several cases no explanation, is that the actual mechanical skill shown by the children—directness of aim, straightness of throw—in these games is very much greater when directed towards skittles which have been previously personified by the child than when the game is a mere game.

Plasticine can also be effectively used to this end.

M.C., Girl, aged 10. While playing shop she began to spring a piece of metal against the side of the shop. Plasticine was suggested as a less dangerous material, and balls of plasticine were thrown hard against the wall. Worker pinned up paper as a target, and asked if she would like to draw anything. She replied "Yes" eagerly and drew a man. She threw balls

---

*Counter-proposals of this kind said in a neutral manner are often made with some children to test the deliberateness of the arrangement that has presented itself.

again with great satisfaction, then pressed balls hard against the face, hand, and stomach of the drawing.

J.D., Girl, aged 5. She was throwing plasticine against a face on the wall. She had been restless, spiteful, and getting out of hand, but was completely satisfied with this form of violence. Her face became smiling as she threw, and she shouted joyfully at a hit. She was determined to demolish the face, but her aim ws very poor.

Horse chestnuts ("conkers") can serve a similar purpose. The following are illustrations taken from notes of private cases (it is difficult to use conkers at the Institute owing to crowding of space):

E.B., Girl, aged 12. She fetched a basket of conkers and began to throw them about the room with a curious two-sided action, asking at each point, "May I throw these here?" or "You're sure it won't break anything?" On being given permission, she usually began by throwing somewhere else. The whole room was littered with conkers, particularly personal parts representing authority—my desk, etc. I pointed out that that was what she thought her parents were doing to her—making a mess of her life as she was making a mess of my room. This was vigorously and enthusiastically received and a very complete mess made. At the end she threw the conkers all over the room, greatly wishing to throw them at me, longing and fearing to do me harm.

B.I., Boy, aged 9. He brought up trees and made a forest with an attacking army among it, a village put up at the side and arranged so that their guns actually shot at somebody. The entire fair and forest, also racecourse people, then the village, and eventually the course, etc., were all destroyed. There was much excitement— conkers thrown at everybody, killing all animals, etc. A ridge of sand and conkers was made down the centre and he pushed his hands roughly through this. A viaduct bridge was built up at the end and destroyed with bombs (conkers).

On another occasion. I was to set up a village all of large houses at one end of the tray with lots of people and all the Danish soldiers (little ones), and make it look nice. He made a very elaborate wood at his end full of soldiers. He then bombed this with conkers, the village first, killing everybody, his own and my people indiscriminately—finally using handfulls of conkers with tremendous energy. As his emotion became unmanageable, I proposed that we should throw at the door instead, which we did for a bit. He then went back again to bombing, and it was noticeable that he put the church up once or twice and specially bombed it. No special discrimination was made between men and women. Ended with violent emotion, throwing as hard as he could.

Other substances can be also used to a similar end.

F.W., Boy, aged 7. While playing with Matador he became very excited. He tore old structures to pieces with force and passion, and danced about the room with the bits in his hands. He took a long piece and beat on the table, then beat himself rather hard, considered a moment, and did it again deliberately. Then he threw the piece down on the table and began constructive work.

R.S., Boy, aged 9. When carpentering he usually hammered the floor and walls, particularly when he was on the floor looking for lost nails. He talked of what would happen if he knocked the house down, but decided he would not, as then he would not be able to come any more.

As the child grows older, combination of active movement with noise tends to gain in content and to combine into rhythm. This can show itself as rhythmic movement of the whole body, or the rhythmic use of instruments, or of a grinder or a mincer tuned to a definite rhythm.

4. *Rhythm.* In the I.C.P. we have always been deeply interested in the use of rhythm for assisting children to find their own emotional centre and regain an harmonious contact with themselves.

In the years 1932 and 1933 lack of space made it impossible to carry on this side of the work, but at the end of 1933 we were able to pick up the threads again.

Rhythm in connection with the playroom is used as a definite therapeutic tool, and forms a department which stands by itself. Children in the rhythm room experiment with the uses of their bodies and with sound. I am indebted to Miss M. Kirschner, rhythm mistress to the Institute, for the following notes:

"Our primary experiment is to find out whether the children have already discovered a convenient means of self-expression or not, either with their own bodies or with an instrument. Sometimes it is possible to distinguish between experiments made to learn more about the instrument, and experiments made to discover possibilities of self-expression inherent in the instrument. Sometimes the making of the experiment in itself is the child's form of expression. When a child has found an adequate means of expression he will continue to use it with considerable persistence. The form the activity takes develops in response to the emotion the child wishes to express. As, for example, a boy when he first came chose the drum, and would play only this instrument, but when his emotions with regard to this instrument were exhausted he chose a whistle instead, and played on it with perseverance, refusing to return to the drum. Another similar example was that of a girl who first danced and then, having apparently exhausted the interest and satisfaction that dancing gave, took to acrobatics and would for the moment dance no more. Later she returned once more to dancing.

"When children express themselves in movement, their activities fall clearly into the following sections: the use of force; the acquisition or display of skill; letting off steam by violent movement; the enacting of a certain character in dancing or by imitation of its characteristics. For instance, they walk like someone, sit like someone, or dance a character they have seen or conceived. In this form their activity borders on acting.

"Music as well as movement can be a direct method for expressing shapeless emotion. In some cases the things so expressed are apparently without ideational content. For example, a boy of eight years, a stammerer, used to play on a mouth-organ and combine with this a kind of dance. Both by his music and his dance he expressed the acts of approaching and retiring from someone; doing so in a friendly and in a hostile manner; being happy and being sad; becoming excited and quietening down again; but he did not seem to have any conscious idea of what he was doing.

"Sometimes the finding of sounds adequate to their strong but shapeless emotion will lead children to the forming of definite images, and the emotion will then take on definite shape. An instance of this was a boy who played aimlessly a few high notes against a background of low ones. He spoke afterwards with enthusiasm of the Hungarian Rhapsody. He played again in a similar manner and said that the sounds were of firing warships. When he again repeated this, he said he was representing a storm at sea, and the distressed ships' wireless signals. Each time the theme developed and followed the stages of shapeless emotion, the same form being repeated and a name or title put to it after it had been played.

"It should be stressed here that by playing the piano is meant not the playing of pieces already taught, nor the teaching of new specially adapted pieces. On the contrary, the piano, although so much more elaborate an instrument than the drum or whistle, is treated as a drum or any of the other instruments—that is to say, as an instrument for the production of sound which is entirely at the child's disposal, and it is for him to discover its possibilities and effects for himself.

"It is natural that some children should expect to be taught, since children of school age attend the Institute. Teaching of this kind is, however, never undertaken. When a child is keen on the accuracy of his effects, he will not be satisfied with a vague reproduction of his musical imagination, but will study assiduously to get exactly what is wanted: songs, rhythms, harmonies, etc., and these in their turn provide him with a knowledge of music, and to a certain extent with instrumental technique.

"This experimentation produces valuable results on the educational side. Children, when allowed this freedom to investigate any instrument, find it easy to concentrate on the means they choose, and they learn *how* to learn things. There have been some astonishing and unexpected results with children who had shown themselves to be unusually restless, but who, after a short period in the rhythm room, applied themselves with endurance and concentration to their chosen medium.

" As a rule there is no difficulty in getting the children to accept this almost 'new' approach towards musical instruments and bodily movement, but in the case of children who have already had music and dancing lessons, there are sometimes difficulties. The more they have 'learned', the less freely they use either music or the body for the purpose of expressing themselves. This is perhaps a natural result of teaching, since the stress has hitherto been laid primarily on exactness in reproducing something already designed, and quite naturally any spontaneous innovation has been met with disapprobation.

"There are two further reasons why the absorbing and learning of set forms seem to prevent children from imagining anything further:

" 1. They are actually told what to like and what not to like, in order to inculcate good taste.

" 2. A form or technique has been given them, when probably there was no need for it.

"We need to know, therefore, whether or not they have been taught before they come to the I.C.P., and, if they have, what that training has been. If they have had training that has really impressed them, we particularly stress our interest in all their *spontaneous* activities, and, if they are not spontaneously active, we introduce them to the idea of characterisation, as it is unlikely that they will have met with this before, except in play. It will on that account, therefore, appeal to them.

"Both music and movement, though free and creative forms of expression, are obedient to strict laws. Any and every form of balance means subordination to the laws of mechanics: the production of satisfactory results in music depends on more or less conscious subordination to the laws of music. In both cases the thing to which obedience is given is impersonal. To get on in music means to become more sensitive to things outside the self—that is, to acquire an easier and more complete subordination to the objective, and to develop a fuller discipline.

"Should the children combine with someone else in their music, beating a drum in time while someone else plays a rhythm, or dancing or skipping in time to another's playing, they have to subordinate themselves to another person. Hereby they experience another person's speed and expression, which is personal to that other person, and they have to identify themselves with it by some reproduction attuned to its rhythm. This, for neurotic children, as soon as they are able to achieve it, forms a most direct and substantial bridge by which they may learn to adapt themselves to the requirements of the social demands made upon them by everyday life."

·   ·   ·   ·   ·   ·   ·   ·

The next two groups of the class play considered in this chapter give expression to emotional impulses and embody states of mind that are usually hidden from adult observation.

5. *Play that is used to express certain very deep emotional states not recognised in ordinary life.* Much that a child feels and desires to know is inexplicable to itself or to the outside observer. A child is aware of its body in a way strange to the adult, and more aware of this than of any other fact. It is natural, therefore, that a child, when driven by any of its deeper and more inchoate desires, should use its body for experiment in the expression of that desire.

Groos recognises the existence of this element in play, when he sets aside a section of his study for "playful experimentation with the feelings "[12] But the section is disappointing in that all the phenomena considered under this head are those of adults, and the only examples given of those mechanisms in children are those of plays with surprise, suspense, and fear, points which we shall consider later (p. 159), but which do not come into this present section.

Permanent elements in this form of play are a child's love of tying up his fellows and being tied up himself, chasing and imprisoning his fellows and urging them to chase and imprison him. It is this motive that underlies much of the delight children find in inventing games of Red Indians, gangsters, and pirates.

The following are extracts from the case-sheets of the I.C.P. illustrating this form of play:

M.E., Girl, aged 13. She grabbed worker, saying, " You be an old witch and run after me and chase me and treat me very badly—come on." The witch put her in her den, but she escaped, and the witch looked for her. When she was found, she said she had taken the witch's magic pennies and refused to say where they were found. She produced a long scarf and said she was to be tied up.

On another occasion. She was playing a game that she was a mother, and worker the elder daughter with a doll baby. The elder daughter was instructed to commit many offences, eating baby's cake, cutting baby's face, and finally trying to run away secretly. The mother returned in time to find this, and attempted to tie up workers violently with great delight—a procedure which was prevented.

A.J., Girl, aged 6. She said, " I am Goldilocks and you are the bear. You catch me and eat me up." I caught her, and she was interested and a little awed by the relish with which I " ate " her, but she enjoyed it and suggested that we should get more children and eat them.

G.W., Girl, aged 13. She tied me up to the curtain with string,* almost hurting my hands, and said I was a prisoner and that she was going to bury me in a grave in the churchyard. She refused to enlarge on this to say what I had done or who I was supposed to be. When she had secured me more or less tightly, she put her arms round my waist and said, " Oh, Ducky." B. (a boy aged 12) came in as a chivalrous knight and attacked her so that I could release myself. It was then time to go home.

J.M., Boy aged 10½. He asked for a game of hide-and-seek, which was played in the dark at his own request.

Another variation of this impulse is the emotional satisfaction given to some children by the assumption of certain bodily positions. In some cases it is a kind of gymnastic attempt to do new strange feats with the body, to endure uncomfortable positions, and here comes in the joy in running, climbing, and wrestling for their own sake and not to achieve particular results, and the physical contortions that many boys deeply enjoy. In other children the adoption of certain positions seems to express an unconscious hunger for some emotional satisfaction which these postures symbolise.

B.G., Boy, aged 12. He was on the floor a great deal, and twice remained perfectly still on his side for several seconds. Worker failed to get his phantasy of what he was doing. The second time she remarked that it seemed a favourite position of his. He replied, " Impertinence ", but later returned to the same position.

Another occasion. When playing statues and acting as a monkey, he lay on his back with his legs in the air, and in doing so repeated an action which is found through all his play. Sometimes he would just lie on the floor without any particular reason for minutes at a time. At others he used the permissive element of football to cover his desire, shooting a goal which he said was the goal which would save the match, and throwing himself on the floor in doing so.

G.W., Girl, aged 13. (She invented this herself.) She lay on the floor, throwing at the skittles overhead, and worker throwing ball back for her to catch. She feigned to be, or was really, afraid of the ball hitting her face, but insisted on continuing the game in this manner.

F.S., Girl, aged 10. She amused herself by refusing all suggestions of apparatus, and wandered round the room, suddenly seizing worker's arm

---

*This procedure is contrary to the rules of the Institute, which do not allow of aggressive acts being carried out in reality against adults. In this case the adult concerned was a visiting physician involved by chance in a group game. The extract is included because it shows the ambivalence of these actions.

or body and attempting to let herself swing, hugging her, and lying on the floor. She handled things on all the tables, then shook herself, saying, " I don't like that " in baby tones.

In the I.C.P., emotion of this kind is directed and given shape in the rhythm room.

It is difficult to discover what kind of child spontaneously develops this type of play, but, for whichever type of child it may be, freedom to express themselves in this way, and a sympathetic reception of their efforts, are prime necessities. As has been pointed out by Dr. H. H. Hamilton Pearson (Physician to the Children's Department of the Institute of Medical Psychology), children can be divided into those to whom physical expression is of main importance, intellectual and emotional expressions taking second place, and those in whom the inter-relation between the basic forms of experience is arranged in other ways. For those children to whom the physical side of life is of primary importance, sympathy with the drive in them to express themselves through physical experience is a matter of fundamental importance to their success and well-being.

The next type of play to be considered is that of Personification in Action, out of which later grows drama.

6. *Personification.* Most children and many adults instinctively like dressing-up. In children this impulse takes many forms.

(a) *Totally shapeless and meaningless " plays "* in which the personification, meaning and action of the children perpetually change—an activity very satisfying to themselves, but bewildering in the extreme to the adult observer. For example:

M.E., Girl, aged 13, and F.V., Girl aged 7.

Enter M.E. and F.V. and wander round. M.E. says something about the wood.

F.V. " It seems to me that this is an enchanted wood."

M.E. says something about a nightingale singing. This is repeated four times. Worker then leaves them for ten minutes, and on her return both girls again come in. M.E. tells F.V. to be a highwayman.

F.V. " Money or your life."

M.E. " Here you are; can you give me change? "

F.V. then becomes a Princess. They sit on stools and M.E. asks the " fair maid " to fetch a drink. They both get a jug and mugs. M.E. pours out, giving F.V. a mug which is said to be dirty, and they both drink. M.E. then collapses and demands water, which F.V. gives her. M.E. nearly chokes but drains the mug.

They then sit on two stools again and sing a love song. M.E. puts F.V.'s head on her shoulder. M.E. suddenly leaps up and tells F.V. she is old and ugly and must leave. F.V. refuses, so M.E. knocks her down and cuts her throat. This, however, does not seem to kill F.V., as M.E. goes on threatening her life for quite a long while.

Or here is another example of this shapeless acting which appeared at the time very satisfying to the actors but was exceedingly confusing to follow. In each case the plays were made up spontaneously by the children, who played alone, but demanded an audience of an adult worker. The characters in the following "story" were also two girls, both aged 11 years.

M.B. and M.C. The details were extraordinarily confusing and the characters changed perpetually. Minnie was the murderer. She stabbed a young lady in the chest and injected poison into her arm. She escaped detection. She then married a "beautiful lady" (Margaret) whom she taught to murder. They then hired a carriage and were driven to the house of an old Jew. They stabbed him and took his jewels. They then went to the neighbour's (Mrs. S—) house and threw the stolen jewels up her chimney. Police (Minnie) came and arrested Margaret, and she was found guilty, having been taken to court before a judge (Minnie), and was then locked in a dungeon. At this point the game ended.

Plays as vague and wandering as these two examples do not occur very frequently among children. They seem to need both a particular temperament and special circumstances for their creation. When, however, they do appear they are carried through by the children who create them with a very curious and striking intensity, and appear to give the actors special and peculiar satisfaction. They are in their shapelessness and poignancy reminiscent of the scenes which pass through the mind of Bloom in James Joyce's *Ulysses,* and have some of the same features that characterise Joyce's imagination.

Sometimes an adult, if sufficiently sympathetic, is included in this type of play, but owing to the mentality of adults, proper participation in a drama of this vagueness is exceedingly difficult, and the play unwittingly begins to take slightly more form.

A very significant variant of this type of roving play is shown when the children take a familiar type of setting and use it to work out their own most intimate phantasies.

(b) *Plays in which children dramatise their own emotions in symbolic form.* Owing to the mutual shyness and suspicion often found between children and adults, this type of play is not so often seen outside institutions such as the I.C.P., and the following extract has been included as a good example in itself, and at the same time as illustrating the use that plays of this kind can be to the child.

K.S., a girl of 12 years, an only child, who was referred to the Institute in 1930 for pilfering, devised the following repetitions of a play made up and acted by herself upon several successive days.

Kristine with ingenuity and imagination dressed herself out of mere scraps as a Princess. Flying cloak, long brown hair tied with blue ribbon, a kerchief, lace hanging from her wrists, finally a long piece of white veiling drawn over her face in the fashion of a bride.

ACT I

The Princess escapes from the palace to the arms of her lover (Alec, part taken by worker), who is waiting in the palace grounds. The Prince gives the signal of escape—an owl's hoot, and a handkerchief waved three times. The Princess is very much afraid of her father.

They fly away together on horseback, but unfortunately are overtaken by the King, and an interview takes place between the King and the Princess. Alec awaits her in the wood where they have been hiding.

ACT II

The Princess steps forward to meet the King, her father (same worker who took the part of Alec in Act I), with gestures befitting a true Princess of royal blood, and with a noble courage and heroism she faces the encounter. The King is angry, and the Princess says she will leave him, never to return. The King pleads with her as a daughter, but the Princess, answering him as " Father ", says she is no daughter of his and never has been. She says that she will now go and live with Alec. As the King pleads, she reminds him of the night he came to her bedroom with a gun to shoot her (this appeared as the chief crime against him). The King queries its happening, but the Princess asserts that it was so, and that it was done from jealousy. The King asks what message she has for her mother. The Princess answers, "Tell her I will meet her by the greenwood tree at eleven to-night."

Throughout, the Princess defies her father (worker) with subdued passion in the voice of a tragedy queen.

ACT III

Meeting between the Princess and her mother (worker).
The Princess shows much affection for her mother and tells her that she too

must escape from the King; that he is the wickedest man in the world—his cruelty and evil know no bounds and he is also an impostor (this has been known to the Princess but not to the mother). The mother agrees to go, but while on their journey the King overtakes them again. This time there is a fight, with shots, and the King is wounded. The Princess finally kills him and jumps on his body—great rejoicings. The Princess and Alec joy dance together.
The play ended.

1st Repetition

Kristine asked if she might do her play again. She collected material from the playroom, her eyes glowing with excitement. The costumes were considered in detail—much the same as last time, with the addition of some silver tinsel which formed anklets, tied with pink bows, and a silver crest on her forehead. Little bows furnished other items of dress. Finally the Prince and Princess were supplied with silk handkerchiefs in their belts.

ACT I

The Princess escapes from the palace in fear of the King.

ACT II. *Flight*

Ovetaken by the King. The Princess goes forward to meet him—duologue here the same—defies the King; no daughter of his, reminds him of the evening he came into her bedroom with a gun to shoot her. She then tells the King that he is an imposter and no King, and this time adds, "You killed my father." He asks how she could have known and she replies, "I listened outside the door and heard the rascal knaves, your servants."

ACT III

Same conversation with mother under the greenwood tree, at eleven o'clock the following night. Affection displayed. Relates the awful secret regarding the King. The King follows and the Princess demands from Alec her pearl gun, with which she shoots the King. He falls dead—she stamps on him. He is still not dead—he is then chloroformed, using a small rubber doll with a hole in the back as puffer.
The Princess then takes Alec to her secret drawer, where she shows him the blood-stained garment belonging to her murdered father, also the rope (a reel of silk) which had been used for hanging judges under the greenwood tree. Much rejoicing, and all the prisoners are released in honour of the occasion, the Princess unlocking the doors herself and saying she is an Italian and Alec an English Prince.

2nd Repetition

The play was acted in the same form and sequence, with certain elaborations of the father theme and change of manner in the scenes with father. In the scene between the father and Kristine, she is not so serious and tragic. Previously she addressed the King with passionate hate, this time in a hoity-toity, almost flippant manner.

She moved round the King, airing her graces in dancing gestures, with little respect for his dignity and none for his authority.

The dialogue here was the same, but she missed out the incident of the King entering her bedroom with intent to kill, and the whole scene was acted in a lighter vein. At the end she took the King to see her father's grave, then recounted the event to Alec with great emphasis.

The scene with the mother was brief, as it was taken by another child, as was also the same scene of the father's death. The King returned and fell to the ground on being chloroformed by Kristine. The other methods of killing were omitted.

The dying King pleaded with Kristine for reconciliation. Kristine accepted this appeal—her emotions changed to pity and remorse that he was dying—she melted, her eyes became sad and almost filled with tears. She wept demonstratively over his dead body.

She would have liked a funeral, but left Alec and the mother to gather flowers while she sought the piano and played a tune. The funeral theme became the dominating factor. She went to the spot where her real father was buried and found that he had disappeared.

This became too much for the other girl, and the scene was hastily turned into a banquet and rejoicings.

3rd Repetition

A doll and much bedding were taken downstairs. The doll was put to bed on a chair and kissed affectionately. The opening scene consisted of a dance by Princess Kristine, who was overjoyed at the prospect of running away with Prince Alec and taking the baby with her.

4th Repetition

She wished to act the same play, but suggested an additional first act in the palace prior to running away: a feast on the King's birthday.

Cast.	Princess	.	.	Kristine.
	Alec	.	.	Worker (female).
	King	.	.	Worker (male).
	Queen	.	.	Jean.
	Baby	.	.	Doll.

A bed was arranged for the baby and it was carefully put to bed behind the curtain. Kristine directed that when the Princess asked for water, the King should reply, "No water." The Princess asked for rice, the King replied, "Yes, but no treacle." The King denied the Princess, and was altogether very hard and dominant and cruel. The Princess took up a martyr-like attitude, became silent, tragic, and refused to eat anything. She retired to her room (the corner of a dark ante-room to the stage), wrapped herself in an old red curtain found there and, huddled in a dark corner, feigned illness. (When discovered, she appeared so completely prostrate, limp, and pallid that she might well have been in appearance extremely ill. She feigned unconsciousness with effective realism.) The kind Queen tried to bring her back to life, told her that her baby wanted her, but she remained unconscious. The doctor was sent for and suggested injections to bring the Princess back to health. She began to wake up as from a horrible dream, dazed and with startled eyes and quick breathing, raised her body spasmodically; refused to stand up. Again the Queen spoke to her of her baby, saying it was crying. The Princess in a voice of command: "Bring him to me." She held the baby in her arms, the gesture completely that of the mother. She remained too ill to get up and said that only bluebell juice squeezed on her eyes could give her complete recovery.

The Princess arose and returned to the stage, where she dressed the baby. Then she made a bed on the stage on which she lay with the baby. She draped the curtain very effectively over her, her arms free in a protective attitude to the child who was placed carefully near to her with its head on the pillow. (Kristine gave the impression that she would have lain there for any length of time, as in the previous feigned illness. She was in no hurry to be discovered or appreciated.)

After this the Princess was a little doubtful as to the course of the play. She finally consented to take some lessons from the royal tutors, such as exercises of a fantastic order in the royal gymnasium.

5th Repetition

Kristine now became the cook, making delicacies for the royal banquet, talking meanwhile in a disparaging way of the Princess and the King who was an impostor.

Characters.				
Princess—Cook	.	.	.	Kristine.
Queen	.	.	.	Jean.
King	.	.	.	Worker (female).
Servant	.	.	.	Winnie.

Grand procession to the banqueting-table. The Princess became the cook who was asked what she meant by saying the King was an impostor. She replied that it was true, that she was going to marry a Prince and would never again have to cook for the King or Queen. She visited the King and Queen as a Princess and stole toy money from the Treasure Chest, which was on the table. She offered to find them a new cook in the person of another worker who had just arrived. The missing money was found in the servant's pocket.

The King asked the Princess to bring the Prince to the palace. She got out of this by staging a hunting accident, and swooned as the imaginary Prince fell from his horse. She recovered after being suitably ministered to by all the characters, and murmured, " It was I who stole that money." She was brought to the palace for convalescence.

6th Repetition

The worker offered herself as lady's maid to the Princess. On the way to the palace, Kristine slipped a coin into the worker's pocket. She then introduced the subject of money stolen from the King's Treasury, and made a search and found it in the maid's pocket.

The King repeatedly asked the Princess to bring the Prince to the palace. Kristine unwillingly agreed. As she went to fetch him, she played the scene of an accident happening to him, and finally fainted in the maid's arms. As she came to, she made a rather dramatic confession that she had stolen the money and put it in the maid's pocket. This fell a little flat. Soon she began violently hunting for the Prince, wishing the maid to prevent her. When she found him, she required the " doctor's " opinion that he would recover and know her again.

Her part as Princess was interchanged with that of cook. When the King stated that his former cook had married a Prince, she did not disagree, but the sequence in her mind was not clear.

7th Repetition

A feast was not introduced to begin with. It occurred on the King's birthday. A baby had already appeared, and had to be put to bed.

A conversation arose with the King concerning food.

At last the reason for the Princess's flight appeared. Previously this was taken for granted, or the reason felt to be too painful for dramatisation.

The Prince had now disappeared. The flight in action from the overbearing father now gave way to flight into sickness. The child dramatised with extreme aptness the real psychological value of illness in these circumstances. The over-bearing tyrant of a father was turned by the daughter's sickness into the solicitous father who with the equally solicitous mother endeavoured to restore her good health. Alec, the bridegroom, had been of use in the first form of the story as an aid to escape, but with the introduction of the baby, and with the new method of flight into illness, he became unnecessary to the central purpose of the drama and disappeared.

In this story the child had taken the familiar background of a fairy-story skeleton, and had used it to work out her own problems. Quite often, however, the children dramatise the story as it is told.

(c) *Representations of known stories in free form.* The following is a play written by a girl of 13, taken from the story of *Anance, the Spider.*

THE STORY FOR A PLAY (*dictated as given here*)

Title: *Anance the Spider of the Large Red Rock.*

There was a famine: nothing to eat at all, not a scrap anywhere (emphatic). The spider Anance was told to go and get something to eat. There was a big red rock, and Anance went to buy some knives; he stuck them up all round the rock, blades up to the sky. Soon a deer appeared; and he said, "Good morning" to the deer. Another deer appeared and said, "Isn't it miserable with nothing to eat at all?" Anance said, "If you come round this rock I'll give you something to eat," and the deer was ever so glad. So he followed Anance, and Anance said, "If you just say, 'What a large red rock', you'll have something to eat." So he shouted out, "What a large red rock." Instantly a huge bird appeared and seized the deer in his mouth and flew up with him a long way. And Anance said, "Drop the deer", so he dropped it, and it fell on the knives, and the wound was so bad that he died at once. Anance dragged the deer home and had him for dinner. And that kept on, and he got so fat. And a wise old rat came along and he was told to do the same; but he pretended to be deaf. So Anance decided to say it for him. Anance said, "Why can't you say, 'A large red rock?'" And as he did so the bird came and picked Anance up. But Anance bellowed out, "It was rat! Rat! Rat!" The bird took no notice and dropped him on to the knives. The rat was so pleased that he ran home to tell the good news. And then the gods sent rain and there was food for man and beast.

This story was later dramatised, and with a mixture of other stories from the same reading book.

Here is another example, also dictated to a worker:

Girl, aged 13, and Boy, aged 9. A Red Indian father and two daughters marooned on an island, one called Adga and the other Amber, the selfish one. Looking for food, father (Bobby) found the skull of an adder, who tells him of a dead boar under a tree. They find this and eat it. One daughter goes out to look for firewood and meets the skull of an adder again, who asks her to marry him. She scornfully refuses him, saying

"Who would wish to marry the skull of an adder?" Then she goes home
and the other girl goes out. The same thing happens, and she says, "I
don't mind if I do." The adder had been so kind in showing them where
the food was. They go and ask the father's consent, he give it, then a gust
of wind comes and blows over the adder, and it arises a handsome Prince.

The girl went over the details several times and was consistent about them.
Then this was acted.

Characters.	Father	.	.	Bobby.
	Amber	.	.	Worker.
	Adga .	.	.	Grace.
	Adder	.	.	Worker.

The adder's father chases Grace, and she is rescued by a new Prince, who
fights the adder's father and kills him, and marries the girl. The corpse of
the adder's father has now to be disposed of. A vague patch . . . ultimately
a rose-tree is planted on him.

The Princess and her husband walk in the wood; she sees the roses and
wants to pick one. The Prince objects, saying he has many more beautiful
things at home, but the Princess insists, gets permission, picks the rose,
pricks her finger, and three drops of blood fall on the adder's corpse and
he comes to life again.

End of play.

ANOTHER PLAY BY THE SAME GIRL

Leah and Blanchette. A grandmother, dying, pulls two candles from under
her pillow, giving them to her two granddaughters. The candles must be
lighted only at night and then a fairy would appear and grant the girls any
wish. Blanchette (Grace) loves her grandmother—Leah does not. The two
girls go for a walk and come to a gate. The bad girl stands on one side and
her sister on the other. A Prince comes along and both the girls attract his
attention. He comes through the gate and chooses the nice girl,
Blanchette. They marry and a few weeks later have a baby.

The bad sister wants the married one's rose-tree to die, out of spite, so she
lights her candle and a witch appears who tells her to whirl a snake three
times round the tree. She does this, and the tree dies. Leah then goes to
the husband, who accepts her as his wife. The baby appears to be left to
her.

(d) *Another variant of this type of play* is the use by children of stock figures
such as pirates, Indians, cowboys, and stories arising out of actual historical
fact, and turning them into running plays which express the children's own
feelings. It is usually the less respectable feelings that are dramatised in this

manner, and thus this classification crosses in several ways that of Group 5. Here are some examples:

C.B., Boy, aged 10, and I.C., Girl, aged 9. C.B. painted his chest with coloured chalk and water, and dressed himself in Red Indian trousers. I.C. and worker were Indians, B.G. (Boy), another worker, and a shy new girl were settlers. C.B. was very active and busy, and full of loud conversation and orders, but they were appropriate, and he was very fair to other people's rights and very reasonable.

They made a tent of a strip of trellis and covered it with things which they fetched from the acting box. A lot of trouble was taken in making and mending the tent. C.B. was proud that this tent was much better than that of the settlers.

I.C. stayed most of the time inside, and worker was posted outside, on guard with a rifle or machine gun. C.B. was fascinated by the noise made for the firing of the machine gun. There was some attacking by the settlers which was actively repulsed, but the chief occupation was collecting weapons and storing them in the tent and keeping the tent mended.

I.C., Girl, aged 9. (Extracts from a report of this child on the same occasion.) She played Indians with C.B. She put a ruler in her mouth, holding it in the centre and prancing about: she pushed me in the back and seized hold of me. Then she "cut off my hand" with a ruler. She hid in the bushes and threw out sticks as arrows at me. With C.B.'s help she killed B.G. and me, suggested stealing our plans and did so herself.

She was very happy and busy all the afternoon and hardly ever left the tent. She spent her time pinning the parts together (which she did thoroughly and well), and arranging the internal things like rugs and beds and weapons. For short periods she lay quietly on her bed. She played the woman completely and well. She asked C.B. if she might come into and share his tent. She conversed and argued with him a good deal on equal terms, and did not hesitate to act on her own, though she did not interfere with his actions, and for the most part accepted his orders and suggestions. She left the tent to fetch hats, which she distributed to us, and jewellery which she stored in the tent with the weapons. Once or twice she rushed out against the settlers who were threatening the tent.

On another occasion. On Red Indians being suggested, she immediately agreed, and said she would make a tent with the dressing-up clothes. She fetched these, and put a paper cap on her head and started with the boys to make the tent. Then she went to dancing. On her return the boys had gone off, but she at once collected them and insisted that the workers should all be cowboys, as the children did not want a grown-up on their side. I.C. wore a wreath on her head. The children armed themselves with sticks, crept up, surrounding the workers, captured them, and shut them up in prison. I.C. said they could not escape, as the only way out was through a den of lions. The lions obeyed the Indians, but would eat the cowboys. She then brought food which was poison, but *she* could eat it and it would not poison her. She went back to her tent. The cowboys said they were hungry and wanted to be let out. She brought "human flesh" for them to eat, and threatened to cut off their heads if they did not eat it (it was cooked). As each cowboy ate it, he was allowed in turn to pass through the den of lions unharmed. On being asked whose flesh it was, she said it was "St. James Albert", and he was killed yesterday, and if the cowboys did not eat it, they would be killed and be "human flesh" themselves the next day.

The cowboys were recaptured and made to eat "lion's flesh" and "lion's blood". It had something in it to make them sleep for twenty years. When one cowboy suggested taking the lower porton, I.C. said that would make him sleep for forty years. The cowboys were then put on "elephants" (C.B.'s idea), and woke up to find themselves on the elephants and all their gold dug up from the ground, and taken by the Indians. They were told to attack the Indians at night, and were beaten. I.C. said the reason of the attack was that the workers saw her, the only woman, go out, so decided to attack the men when they were alone. I.C. returned disguised as a bear, and then the cowboys found she was a woman. When told there were only ten more minutes, the children decided to end by a final execution, and I.C. brought a stone slab on which to cut off heads. The stone was too heavy to hold, so each in turn had to put his head over a low door and have it sawn off by I.C. and another boy with sticks.

(*e*) *Another variant of spontaneous drama* is the little running plays made up by children about current events; but as these come more properly in the class of play that is concerned with a child's relationship to its environment, consideration of them will be postponed to a later chapter.

(*f*) *Finally we come to full co-ordinated acting of plays with a set text*, such as is done in many schools, where the text is either written by the children, as in the Russells' school[24], or by an adult writer for children. But as the discipline of carrying out pre-arranged plans does not come within the scope of the work of the Institute, examples of this form are not included. Here we cross the border-line between play and artistic creation, and find ourselves outside the scope of our enquiry. There is, however, one more phenomenon which must be referred to, and which comes most properly within the scope of this chapter, and that is the phenomenon of ritual.

RITUAL

Ritual is a characteristic which recurs throughout children's play and is included here, as it most usually occurs in connection with movement. In the life of all primitive peoples, and in the religious life of almost all people, there occurs from time to time ordered and repetitive performance of well-defined acts in a definite sequence. This is equally true of children. One explanation of this happening, when it occurs in children, is that a thought process is at work in a deeper layer of the mind which has a real sequence in the region in which it is active, analogous to the sequence of logic, but which, being unable, or unwilling to express itself in words, throws itself into concrete expression in a series of apparently unconnected symbols. To the eye of the observer the hidden logic does not appear, and there appears instead a meticulous repetition in a fixed order of apparently meaningless acts. All children, as their games—and particularly the traditional games–most strikingly show, have a tendency to originate spontaneously and to demand from others a curiously fixed ritual. Any collection of children's games will give abundant evidence of this peculiarity, and a very long chapter could be written on the part that ordered ritual plays in the lives and development of little children.

In the neurotic child, ritual shows itself in two ways:

1. By the child developing a series of acts which it is necessary for it to perform in more or less the same order, before it is able to settle to work or play.

2. In the emergence of a certain set order of events *in* the child's play, an order which, once having fixed itself, forms a framework within which developing ideas can allow themselves to show change and progress, but without which the child cannot play at all.

Records of the first type of ritual among the Institute children are hard to produce satisfactorily, for the early repetitions are rarely recognised and so not adequately described, and the ritual, once noticed, tends to be described in future in terms too cursory for effective quotation. For example:

F.H., Girl, aged 2. She agreed to play water games, and asked for a flannel, scrubbing-brush, and mat, and started to wash the floor with all the usual ritual.

On another occasion. She was provided with water on arrival, and attempted to play with it, but very soon started the usual ritual of washing the floor. This seems to be a compulsive action. She tried to join worker in other games, but gradually became absorbed in her floor and washing until another child joined her at the water tray. All her energy was then concentrated on trying to prevent the other girl from having anything to play with.

On another occasion. On arrival she was provided with water, and immediately set to work upon her floor-washing ritual. After ten minutes another girl joined them, and, although F.H. continued washing for a while, her interest in it evaporated. For the first time she omitted the last act, viz. to lay paper over the part she had cleaned and request me not to step on the clean wet floor.

On another occasion. When she arrived she said, " I'm not going to wash the floor to-day." She therefore sat down with another girl and began threading cubes, being just a little careful as to which half were hers and which belonged to the other. Shortly afterwards, dry sand was provided and a little water, and almost at once she said, " I'd better wash the floor," and demanded the wherewithal, getting excited and impatient until it was provided. The last stage of the ritual was again completely omitted, and the whole thing ws performed with much less earnestness than usual. She was a little annoyed when the other child wiped a bit of the floor which she had not finished, but there was no tension nor anxiety.*

Certain children show an almost uncanny predisposition for the instant-aneous development of ritual, as the following extract shows:

R.C., Boy, aged 5½. He thought he would like to paint, and the material was collected; it then appeared that he had no experience of what to do. He drew a dryish brush over a paint and then across the paper and made no mark. Worker took the brush, dipped it in water, and rubbed it across a cake of red paint in one box, and, as that colour did not come off, across a similar colour in another box. This came off well, and worker handed it back to him.

He immediately adopted this as a ritual, and for the next quarter of an hour or so, irrespective of requirements, dipped the brush full into the water, drew it over the hard red in one box, lightly touched the same red in the other box, and so to a to-and-fro movement across the paper. This was repeated without a break or alteration.

The following series of a worker's notes taken of a girl of six show a curious variety of this type of ritual.

R.A., Girl, aged 6. She took up an animal and chased me, then, at her suggestion, I chased her with the animal. We ate each other up, etc. Next we made a house, with chairs and tables, behind the door-curtains. She

---

*At the discussion following this lecture, a member of the audience quoted a child at her infant school who had been washing for a month, and other girls who must wash floors for weeks. Also another child who could not go to sleep until her room was arranged like a dormitory, with three beds. Another member of the audience quoted children playing out rituals with puppets, and also referred to the story of the sand pile in *Aspects of Child Life and Education.*

brought in eleven bowls of water. We washed and polished the house, spilt water, and wiped it up. R.A. drank a lot.

1st Repetition. We played house, putting chairs and tables round the fire, and she brought in seven jugs of water. We went through a day, starting by getting up in the morning and finishing by going to bed. This was punctuated by going to the lavatory twice and drinking.

2nd Repetition. Played house again. Four jugs of water brought in. We went through part of the day; this was punctuated with going to the lavatory twice, then a hunting game. I was naughty and she hit me, and then drank.

3rd Repetition. Played house. Six jugs of water, punctuated by looking out of the window at birds, etc. Lavatory twice. Jumping down stairs. Drinking.

4th Repetition. Played house. Two jugs of water and two bowls of peas, punctuated by hunting, lavatory twice, jumping down stairs. She hit me, and did some sweeping and deliberately spilled water. Then she drank.

Here is another example of ritual play spontaneously developing out of experience:

G.T., Boy, aged 6. He got out Kliptiko and began making his single-line track. He made out my privilege pass and I bought tickets for a lady and a little boy. We began our journey from Leighton Buzzard. No mishaps. He began making a branch line, forgetting all about the journey. He continued to fiddle with the metal line. Occasionally he told me what conversation to make: "Tell your little boy that you recognise all these stations"; "Tell your little boy you wonder why you are stopping; then put your head out of the window and you see the engine has been taken off"; "Tell your little boy that you hear a train coming, but you can't see one, and you are very surprised to see one coming round the corner"; etc.

1st Repetition. He began immediately to write out my "privilege pass", then gave me tickets. I then drew his attention to the station having disappeared. He was very much amused and immediately got out Kliptiko and made the rails. Then he forgot the trains and had to be reminded. Suddenly he thought he would like a tunnel. This he made with large wooden bricks and a slate; after which he made a platform, a signal-box, and level-crossing gates. This occupied so much of his attention that he forgot all about the journey—it took me one and a quarter hours to reach Warwick Avenue. He told me that my little boy was to say that he didn't like going through tunnels.

2nd Repetition. He played the usual journey from Leighton Buzzard to Warwick Avenue. He and his mother had missed all their connections. In my journey I had to miss all my connections; in addition, my train went no further than to Baker Street. I was not to notice it and to return to Regent's Park, and also was to pass Warwick Avenue and to go on to Maida Vale, from where I had to make the very tedious journey back to Warwick Avenue. He built a tunnel and station, as previously, and all the usual routine of "privilege pass" and tickets had to take place.

3rd Repetition. He immediately got down Kliptiko and began to make his rails. He said he was not going to make a station and tunnel to-day, as it took up so much time, and we had to take them to pieces at the end. He preferred that we should make the complete return journey to and from Leighton Buzzard. He told me he had a good idea to-day. He was going to give me a wrongly dated pass and I would have to pay 7 shillings on it (this had happened to his mother in October). I pretended I had not 7s. on me, so he said I must pay as much as I could and I could pay the balance next month.

In some ways this compared with the Princess drama given earlier.

A child's choice of material is sometimes regulated by the same tendency to ritual. Some children must always do one thing first, some another; some are faced by an inner necessity each afternoon to use their material in the same order and to express with it a similar sequence of ideas. Examples:

B.C., Girl, aged 5. She made a rectangular pattern with mosaics. Then she made a man with a different kind of mosaic. She then went to the water room. She said she wanted to play with fish. She put them into the water, but then took the toy lavatory and poured water from one vessel to another and then into the lavatory. Then she went to dancing. After dancing she went to the sand tray and made a world with tiny people, animals, and transport. The red fire-engine was in the middle and the red fire-escape against the outer wall. Then she began to play with sand, using a small bowl at first, and making pies, but the vessels chosen became bigger and bigger until at last she used the saucepan, throwing the sand about in large heaps. Water was added; she showed increasing satisfaction as the sand grew wetter, lifting lumps of it and splashing it into pools.

On another occasion. She accepted mosaics eagerly, and made first a straggling pattern, which was re-arranged until it became square. She was not satisfied with this, but broke it up and made a pyramid design. She then went to the lavatory. She demanded plasticine and made a grotesque figure—a man with a very round head and body, and legs coming out of his neck. Then with much laughter she hammered him flat. Worker opened a new packet of sand and gave her half, but she wanted all. The sand was wetted and dropped about in large lumps.

It is an open question what exactly we are observing here. How far is this tendency to shape actions into repetitive order common to sick and to normal children? How far is it an inherent human trait and how far a manifestation of morbidity? Is it to be encouraged, or should efforts be made to help the child develop a freer relationship to its own mental processes and to the material? How far is this phenomenon a common one among all children?

In the discussion that followed the lectures that form the kernel of this book, some of these questions were answered in part, instances being cited of normal children playing out rituals with puppets and other plays. From these and the number of other instances that seemed to spring to the minds of the audience in relation to normal children, it seems reasonable to assume that ritual is sufficiently common in normal children to be in no sense in itself a trait of morbidity. Not sufficient data are at present forthcoming to conclude whether it occurs more frequently among normal children than among emotionally disturbed children, nor at which age it is most frequent.

Many children throughout their childhood make magic rituals which they keep entirely to themselves, but which they carefully carry out in daily life in the belief that the performance of them does actually bring about changes in the external world. A. A. Milne in his children's poems[25] gives charming instances of this habit, and most mothers will be able to provide many examples from experiences of their own children.

CHAPTER IV

PLAY AS REPETITION OF EXPERIENCE

"In 1879 Dr. K. Lange urged that a six-year-old child has learned already far more than a student learns in his entire university course. 'These six years have been full of advancement, like the six days of creation.' Concrete conceptions have been accumulated in vast numbers, and the teacher must not assume that a *tabula rasa* is before him."

G. STANLEY HALL.[13]

IN RECENT YEARS much attention has been given to the experiences children pass through in the first year of life, and, owing to the findings of psycho-analysis, more and more importance comes to be laid on these first months of life. Throughout the work of the older observers scattered observations of children in their first two years can be found, but these are not in any sense exact observations, and it is to Bechterew, Charlotte Bühler, and Gesell on the one hand, and the psycho-analytic group on the other, that we are indebted for the beginning of an exact knowledge of this period.

Both Bechterew and Gesell have made attempts to create tests for infancy which could be used in a manner comparable to the tests employed in psychological laboratories for older children, and their aim has been so to arrange the surroundings of the test that the child could be observed undisturbed by the presence of an adult. There are objections to this method, in that a child playing by himself with standardised objects in the centre of a large room is not a child in normal surroundings, and we do not know whether the child himself would choose these types of objects to play with which are provided for him were he able to make his own choice.

It is to Charlotte Bühler[22,23] that we owe the first attempt to observe children scientifically in *their own* environment and to make statistical use of these observations. The method that she and her assistants employed was that of uninterrupted systematic observation of one and the same child under conditions which are normal in his everyday life. A given child was watched, whether waking or sleeping, over a period of twenty-four hours by trained observers, who relieved each other at eight-hour intervals. These observations in no way disturbed the normal daily plan either by day or night. An accurate record in this way was kept throughout the whole twenty-

our hours, and the precise time and duration of every new occurrence
noted. In all, 69 children in the first year of life, including a minimum of five
infants in each month, were observed in this way. Of these, 40 per cent were
children from private homes, and 60 per cent "institution" children. By
children from private homes" is meant, first of all, those children who
were observed in their own home environment, and, secondly, those
children who came to the *Kinderübernahmsstelle* with their mothers. The
remainder were largely children who came to spend a three-week
quarantine period in the *Kinderübernahmsstelle* before being placed in some
institution. With the exception of the "new-born" group (consisting of four
children from one to ten days of age), five complete observations were
always made in each age-group. All children were examined medically
before the investigations were begun, and only healthy babies were selected.

It is clear, as Bühler states, that a preliminary step to the organisation of
his method of work must be an agreement between those who are to
undertake the observations as to points which are to be observed.

With the exception of those of sleep and of suckling, the points chosen by
Dr. Bühler refer in the main to social rather than physiological phenomena,
and are, on the whole, qualitative and quantitative analyses of behaviour.
These and the time analysis of the child's day led her to an endeavour to
establish levels of development for the first year of life. It is regrettable that
no attention has been paid in these studies to the children's reactions to their
baths, their handling, or their toilet training. It is to be hoped that some day
this defect may be remedied.

As this aspect of life has not interested Gesell or Bechterew either, we are,
to date, without any objective studies of it.

We are indeed on the whole without any very exact observations of
children's reactions to their physiological experiences during the first year
of life. In a recent book[27] Dr. Wallon of the Sorbonne has drawn attention to
the marked difference shown in co-ordination between the aimless bodily
movements of the infant and the extraordinarily exact co-ordination of
voluntary and involuntary muscular movements involved in the act of
suckling. He is more interested in the child's attempts to establish a
relationship between itself and the outside world than in the emotional
colouring of these movements.

Professor Bühler[23], in reviewing the kinds of movements made by very
young infants, writes:

"All the periods in which positive or negative movements of expression
were observed, irrespective of whether they were the dominating factor
or just different ways of behaviour (experimenting, single movements,
reception of food), are here grouped together according to time and
contrasted with each other. *We can state concerning them that positive
expressions appear much later than negative ones, and that, although at first they*

are far less than the negative, they finally exceed them considerably during the first year [my italics].

She includes the following table to illustrate this very important observation:

THE DURATION OF OBSERVED POSITIVE AND NEGATIVE
EXPRESSIONAL MOVEMENTS (IN MINUTES)

Age	Positive expressional movements	Accessory Pos. Exp. movements	Total	Negative expressional movements	Accessory Neg. Exp. movements	Total
0·0	—	—	—	104	—	104
0·1	1	—	1	232	—	232
0·2	2	10	12	187	—	187
0·3	3	29	32	179	—	179
0·4	1	32	33	171	—	171
0·5	2	92	94	159	—	159
0·6	4	201	205	122	—	122
0·7	2	223	225	146	—	146
0·8	7	222	229	99	8	107
0·9	10	218	229	83	10	93
0·10	7	264	271	101	2	103
0·11	11	306	317	57	10	67
1·0	11	300	311	77	21	98

Summing up this table, Charlotte Bühler writes:

"The spontaneous reactions include two groups: aimless movement and impulsive sounds in one group, experimenting and lalling in the other. The aimless movements increase in frequency with the decrease of the negative movements, *which have reached their maximum daily value in the first month* [my italics]. They decrease in that moment when the observed experimenting movements begin to broaden. Experimenting, which fills 11 per cent of the waking of a two-year-old, occupies 63 per cent of the waking time of a one-year-old.

Both these observations—that is to say those concerning the negative movements and those concerning experimenting—are of very great importance in connection with the form of play to be described in this chapter.

Concerning the general development of the first year, Professor Bühler writes:

"The maximum periods of dozing, of negative reactions (movements and expressional movements), and of aimless movements grow shorter and shorter; the periods of experimenting and lalling grow always longer. The perseverance of the *one-year-old who spends an uninterrupted two hours and twenty-three minutes in experimenting is especially remarkable* [my italics]. We can also find a great progress in perseverance during the last quarter of the first year. If we measure the various groups of behaviour according to time, we would find: decrease of sleep, increase of waking, lessening of quiet waking, especially of dozing; decrease of negative, increase of positive and spontaneous reactions; growth of positive expressions—a general increase in positive and active behaviour.

We are, then, according to Charlotte Bühler, in possession of three facts with regard to the first year of life:

1. Negative reactions predominate over positive in the first weeks of life, and reach their maximum daily expression in the first month of life.
2. Negative reactions decrease in direct relation to the increase of actions of experiment.
3. Actions of experiment are to be found as early as the second month, and by one year an infant's capacity for concentration has already reached remarkable dimensions. This observation is particularly valuable in its contradistinction to the view generally held concerning infants.

With regard to the second year of life we have very much less information—a few studies of this period occur in Professor Bühler's *Kindheit und Jugend*[26]; and some in Professor Bridges' analysis of the preschool child[28], but no exhaustive study of the phenomena of this year of life is yet available.

To summarise our knowledge of the first two years of life, it would seem that children's experience in these years can be grouped into the following classes:

1. Experiences of movement. Here is included the " Function Play " of Charlotte Bühler to which reference has already been made in Chapter III.
2. Experiences of sensation. Here are included experiences of sight, sound, smell, touch, and taste.
3. Experiences of emotion within the self, attraction towards, repulsion from, and flight from, other phenomena (indicating the experience of fear).
4. Intellectual experiences; experiences of recognition and understanding.
5. Delight in experiment with available phenomena; in this case mainly its own body.
6. Gradual apperception of outside objects and persons. In this process all the above experiences (1–5) will be blended.

We have abundant evidence in the mass of work that has been done on this subject that Groups 1 and 4, and such parts of 5 and 6 as are applied to impersonal objects, have received full recognition from the outside world. When children are exercising these functions they have not only the joy of the exercise itself, but also the deep satisfaction of finding themselves the object of absorbed and serious contemplation on the part of the adults in their world.

As regards Group 2, some of the experiences which come under this head are apt also to become the focus of adult observation, but the ban which we noted in the older observers as covering many aspects of child life (see p. 26) is powerfully operative here, and we are indebted entirely to the psycho-analytic group for such knowledge as we have of this side of a child's experience.

A child's joy in movement in infancy and later childhood has already been considered in Chapter III, and some aspects of his relation to these experiences. A child's inner valuations of those of his experiences which come under Group 3 are very hard to obtain, and we must again thank the psycho-analysts for most of the knowledge that we have of this aspect of early life.*

As regards the experiences of Group 4, the child's reactions in play to some of these will be considered partly in this chapter and partly in Chapter VII.

Upon the study of Group 6 the attention of the educational psychologists have been mainly concentrated.

We ourselves now need to consider part of Group 5 and part of Group 6.

Now, concerning this material which composes much of what would come under Group 6, and some of that coming under Group 5, we are in a curious position. In the latter half of the nineteenth century, child psychologists, much influenced by Wordsworth and his group, and too intimately descended from philosophers, were unable to see children without bias. *Vide*, for example, the author of the story of Roswitha[29,30], who considered the practical details of a child's toilet unfit to come within the sphere of observations of a cultured adult or research worker.

But, if the whole gamut of an infant's day be considered, it will be seen that many things occur to the infant which would properly come under Group 2, and which so far no observers have included in their categories of observation.

Every infant is washed daily and toileted (hair-brushing, nose-cleaning, etc.). He both performs excretions and is the object of attention with regard to them, but so far no detailed study is available of an infant's reactions to these experiences, and, moreover, they are the experiences that most quickly and thoroughly come under the ban of cultural training.

*See Bibliography to Introduction, Section 4 (c).

Observation of the ordinary life and play of ordinary children suggests, however, that the point of view of the adult in regard to these sides of a child's life is not at all the point of view of the child, but that, on the contrary, a very real interest in this side of life exists in every normal child. Susan Isaacs, in her study of *The Social Development in Young Children*[31], quotes many instances of such interest as occurring among her children of from two to six years old. For example, she writes:

"*19.11.24.* At lunch the children had a conversation as to what people were 'made of', and spoke of people being made of pudding, pie, potatoes, coal, etc., and of 'bee-wee', 'try', 'do-do', 'ah-ah', 'bottie'.

"*24.11.24.* The children were getting water to drink in cups, and Harold told the other that he had given Frank some 'wee-wee water' to drink. He often says, 'there's wee-wee water in the bowl' in which he washes his hands. Later he said he had drunk 'wee-wee water', and that the water in the cups was that.

"*26.11.24.* When marching round, the children took the enamel bowls to use as drums; then they put them on the floor and sat in them, first calling them 'boats,' and then as lavatories to 'try' in; Harold and Paul sat in them, saying, 'I'm trying.'

"Paul told Mrs. I., 'Do you know what I have to make me try? Grapefruit.'

"At lunch, Harold said to Mrs. I., 'You are made of try.' Frank, 'You are made of water.' Benjie, 'Of bee-wee.'

"*11.2.25.* After lunch, Frank and Dan made a 'house' with chairs. Frank said, 'And we'll have a little lavatory, a little lav-lav.' Presently he went to the real lavatory, saying, 'Shall we go to our little lavatory?'

"*24.4.25.* Theobald poured water into the sand and called it 'bee-wee sand'.

" Frank was heard to say to another child, 'Shall we put some fæces in a cake and give it to Dan's mummie—and then she won't know what she is eating?' On another occasion he was heard to tell Dan, 'Pass all you have in your bottie.' Dan replied, 'Then I shan't have any more to pass out.' Frank: 'Then your bottie will be flat.'

"*24.1.27.* In their play after lunch, Jane, Priscilla, Jessica, and Dan played a family game which included sitting on 'potties', 'passing fæces', and falling off pots (cushions) with laughter. They went on with this until Mrs. I. called them to come and do something else.

"*24.3.25.* While the others were modelling, for a time Paul, Frank, and Harold had the rugs round them and first ran about as 'fairy godmothers', and then crouched on the platform, each with a rug covering him right over, as 'gramophones', and sang songs, singing, 'Hey diddle diddle', 'Humpty dumpty', and 'bim-bom', 'bee-wee', and 'try-pan'."

Here is a similar story (privately contributed) from the play of a perfectly normal little girl:

> "A child of 3½, playing with her tiger, brought him one day into the drawing-room and sat him end upwise on a cane-seated stool. When asked what he was doing, she said he was doing his 'big'. After sitting him there for some time, she said he was finished. She very carefully wiped his bottom, and then proceeded in play to wipe up the ground underneath the stool.
>
> "This same child, when there was any difficulty in getting her to perform her daily excretions, could always be persuaded to do so by being told that, 'Tiger has gone into the garden to do his "big".' When this was said, Jane immediately retreated to perform the same operation herself with good grace."

To the small child, all parts of its day are interesting, and, although it will learn early not to mention or perform certain parts of its daily routine publicly, it is inevitable that the interest in those events will continue, and will tend to be carried over into play.

In respect of many experiences grouped under Group 2, some of Group 3, and much of Group 5, the child finds himself in the same position. The adult's point of view and the child's vary so greatly about the situations covered by these groups, that the child is confused with regard to them; the battle between adult disapproval and interior delight is so intense that in many cases none of the experiences of these groups comes to light at all.

Now Freud has put forward the proposition that there is a repetition compulsion in all human beings which drives them to repeat in actuality, or in symbol, experiences they have already passed through, whether painful or pleasurable. Whether this is true as a universal law or not, it does seem to be undeniable that small children have a very strong and essential wish to reproduce their own experiences in play, and very early experiences are no exception to this rule.

There seems to be a strong inner drive in all human minds to externalise themselves, or to re-create their experiences in order to be able to assimilate them, and the small child in relation to its early experiences is no exception to this rule.

If allowed to take place at the proper time "unobserved"—or, more exactly, unreproved—and in circumstances which offer many and varied interests, such play is played through and disappears of its own accord as the small personality develops and life affords more interesting emotional outlets. But tacit permission of this kind is rare, and, if it is not given, if opportunities for such play are not forthcoming, or if play of this kind and interest in this side of life meet with too severe a prohibition, this interest tends to become hypostasised, as it were, to undergo no development, and to remain as a fixed image in the deeper layers of the mind. The excretory jokes of adult comic papers, the excretory references and gestures in much music-hall and film comic art, show how this element continues right through into adult life (see p. 8).

As an example of this sort of play, we can take the following extract from Institute case records of a boy of six years old, who was referred for treatment on account of lying and stealing.

R.L., Boy, aged 6. A very small contracted child with lashes much darker than his hair. He looked round the room, peeped into the playroom " shop ", and asked if he might go to the water. He played with a good many of the water toys, but enjoyed most seeing a swan caught in, and driven under by, a fierce stream of water from the tap. Then he put a wet toy on the shelf and it dripped on to the floor. He said with animation that it was " wee-weeing ".

On another occasion. With another boy he played with ducks and fish, filling the sink full of water and putting in all the ducks and fish they could find. He took out some rubber toys, and I showed him how they could squirt. Both boys squirted with zest for a while, then the other left. We now had an orgy of squirting. All the animals " wee-ed " over and over again. They " wee-ed " over each other and over the walls, they were called " dirty things ", they made rude noises, and " did by mistake ". We decided that this was a good joke; then he made them " wee " into his face with great delight, telling them to do it. He took a doll out of the cupboard and said, " She has just come out of an egg."

Playing out themes of this kind does not *encourage* or develop interest in excretion. By allowing escape to an already existent and pent-up interest, which, because it is pent-up, causes neurotic manifestations in other ways, play gives vent to the original interest and, at the same time, brings about an amelioration of the neurosis.

When it is freely allowed, excretory play forms a very important part of the life of small children, and is of considerable significance in their healthy development. It will reappear with persistent regularity in the play of older children who have been without this permissive freedom in early years, if they later come into circumstances where such play is permitted. Such play falls into three categories:

A. Play in which dolls—objects temporarily made into dolls—and sometimes in phantasy the adult playmate, are made to carry out the toilet and excretory performances that the small child itself does.

B. Plays in which the child himself repeats in symbol or in exaggerated mimicry parts of his similar experience.

C. Derivative play, or play which is essentially experiment with all the separate parts of infantile experience.

Instances of play of the first kind occur in Otto Ernst's studies of his own daughter Roswitha, as, for example, in the daily experience of hair-combing:[29]

" Most remarkable is it that, when Roswitha sets to work to dress her children, she opens proceedings by combing their hair (she dislikes her own hair being done). . . And the indignation of the wee mother because ' big girls ' like Ursula and Hedwig scream when they are being dressed! It is still odder, that when my turn comes, and I behave beautifully under the combing process, and labour under the delusion that I shall go up one in mother's estimation, mother, on the contrary, shows great dissatisfaction.

" 'Oh, no, daddy, oo mus' skeam too ', she exclaims, evidently most disappointed and annoyed.

" I screech, consequently, like a torpedo-boat, and am convinced of the fact that even such good children as Roswitha think naughtiness much more interesting than goodness."

Susan Isaccs[31] also quotes many examples of the same kind of play in her observations of normal children.

Apart from play that reproduced the ordinary toilet processes of the day (as with Roswitha above), repetitive play in relation to a child's elementary physiological experiences may, if repetitive play with the senses be excluded, be divided into three groupings:

1. *Play in connection with the mouth.*

The following examples can be taken from Mrs. Isaacs's observations:

" *22.10.24.* George again put the rugs into his mouth when resting. He always puts his plasticine into his mouth.

" *8.5.25.* George and Christopher were sitting opposite each other at one table doing plasticine, and somehow excited each other very much. They began throwing the plasticine at each other, putting it in their mouths and biting it and laughing in an excited, screaming way."

And here are examples of Institute children:

S.P., Girl, aged 4½. She suddenly began to build by placing bricks on me (worker), first on my leg, and then on my head. This was followed by wanting to build in my mouth. She ordered me to put a brick in my mouth. I showed her the brick was too big, and she seized one of the half (red) blocks and held it between her teeth. I said I would build a " mouth ", and did so. This did not satisfy; she merely enjoyed knocking it down.

E.J., Girl, aged 3½. Playing with plasticine, her idea was to make " pies " and " puddings ". She told me to make several things, and insisted that a little boy in plasticine should have teeth and a tongue.

A.J., Boy, aged 5. He started with filling vessels from the big can, and almost immediately he began to snatch at the water with his lips. It was difficult to see whether he drank any or not, although the desire was there. He repeated this drinking gesture several times, but soon passed on to the thought of solids. He took the contents of the water box out, piling them into the water tray, almost obliterating the water. He showed an interest in the contents of the box, asking what they were, putting the ducks back in the water, and then into his own mouth.

Older children who have been inhibited in early youth in play of this kind tend also, when provided with suitable opportunities, spontaneously to improvise similar forms of play.

B.G., Boy, aged 9. (Intellgience Quotient 126). He found a doll's feeding-bottle on the mantelpiece and immediately put it into his mouth. He filled it at the tap, and found the water did not come fast enough through the teat, so he took it off. He filled his bottle several times from the tap, and then washed out the sink. He then pulled the teat off the bottle with his teeth and said he had swallowed it—he chewed it for 10–15 minutes. Worker asked if he was still chewing it and he said, " Yes, I brought it up again." He then said he would play guessing games with worker, and during this game said he had had enough of the teat. He put his hands to his mouth, gave a mighty cough which really appeared to be getting something out of his throat, and spat out the broken teat. He then began to do Decroly tests, during which he whistled or sang loudly all or most of the time. He chewed the wood off the pencil and finally spat it on the floor. Went to the lavatory . . . He found the water-squirt and puffed air into his mouth. Worker asked what that would do, and he said what sounded like " Murder". Worker repeated the question, but he would not say anything further. He filled the squirt in a basin of water at the sink, having first washed out the basin. Then he brought a basin of water into the playroom. He continued to suck the squirt, and also put the whole of the ball end in his mouth. He squirted hard into his mouth and said it was like pumping up a tyre. Part of the time, when sucking, he threw his head right back. He said he wondered whether he could use up all the water in the basin. He said it made him out of breath to drink, and, when asked if it always did so, he said, " Yes, and if I drank more it would kill me." Later he found sand was coming out of the squirt. This he got the squirt to suck up again, and then squirted the sand into his mouth, and, biting a piece of sand with his teeth, asked, " Are my teeth clean?" He squirted the water in the air and said it was "The King's Fountain". He wanted to empty the basin and fill the squirt with dry sand. When told he could go, he went over to the fire and stayed till he was told he must go, trying to bite the paint off the painted animals on the mantelpiece. He went to the lavatory, remarking it was the third time.

The *motif* of suckling, it should be noted, occurs strongly in the above extract, in both active and passive aspects, and is a fairly common component of play. For example:

F.H., Girl, aged 2½. A doll, a nest of boxes, and a Russian nest of dolls were put on a table. She immediately took up the rag doll, set herself down at the table with the doll held to her, and began to rock backwards and forwards with it in an obvious nursing attitude.

On another occasion. She played with the dolls. Worker had a doll; she had a doll. We had to feed them with acorns, but really she held hers and rocked it right up to her breast, and then gave it an acorn. Worker had to do the same, being told to hold it just so in both arms.

M.T., Girl, aged 3. She filled a feeding-bottle at the sink and gave "milk" to the doll after tasting it herself. She found the water did not really come out of the bottle, struggled to get the teat off, could not, so gave it to the worker, saying, "Get the titty off." Then she poured water all over the doll and worker, saying, "Look, your skirt is all wet." After drinking from the bottle, she urinated, and was fascinated with the flush and chain. She washed her hands, asking for both taps to be turned on. She then played with the lavatory basin for some time, emptying and filling, and would not return to the playroom. Worker fetched water toys, duck and fish, and suggested using the sink as there was no room in the basin. She came reluctantly, but enjoyed the sink, and played with the rubber duck, squirting in worker's face. Then she filled the bath, and sucked water from it through a narrow tubing; worker suggested blowing down the tube instead of sucking (the bath was rusty, and the sink had sand and flour in it). She very much enjoyed the big bubbles and the noise. She went upstairs to tea, but returned to the sink, and asked for funnel but did not use it. She asked worker to taste "nice water" through tube. After trying to reach the tap, she asked worker to lift her, and played for a long time with the tap, though held in a most uncomfortable position with no rest for her feet. Urinated again, and played with lavatory basin. She was fascinated by the hot tap, and the water coming straight at her. She refused to leave when someone else wished to come in, saying, "No, I want to stay; turn the taps on!" Worker blew bubbles in the water through a tube. She came closer to watch, then asked to be lifted to reach the tap. She then played with the tap for about five minutes, forgetting her grievance, then got down, dried her hands, and went upstairs on all fours.

Most children have had the experience of being sick—that is, the reversal of the intake of food—when, without anything definite being done by them, something from inside them suddenly comes up through the mouth, accompanied by new taste experiences, and is vomited with force.

R.D., Boy, aged 5½. He poured water into a hole in a rubber dog and squirted the water out upwards, becoming very excited. His attention was called off to another dog. He filled its mouth with water and squirted it out. He then put the policeman in the jar and drowned him.

M.B., Girl, aged 8. She was making pies and had nearly finished, and told me what she was going to do afterwards: "Wash my hands, do up my shoes, find paints and paper and draw with my pencil. It's quite a new one." She then poured water on the remains of the dough, making a sticky semi-liquid mess, which she rubbed all over her hands with evident enjoyment, saying, "It reminds me of sick." Worker asked, "Does if feel nice?" M.B.: "No, not nice; it's horrid, but I like it."

On another occasion. While using mosaics she coughed once. Then, holding her hand to her mouth with fingers bent to form a trumpet, she blew through her fingers with short puffing breaths. Worker asked her if her hands were cold. She replied, "No, I'm making myself sick."

Mrs. Isaacs[31] gives similar examples:

"*10.12.26.* The children (Jane, Conrad, Dan) were playing 'ship', and each child had a waste-paper basket of his own as a 'lavatory'. They pretended to be sick, to make water, and to pass fæces, saying, 'Mine's full', 'Empty it in the sea', and so on.

"*11.12.25.* One of the children brought to school a rubber mouse that could be used as a squirt. They said it 'makes bee-wee out of its mouth.'"

2. *Play connected with the experience of urination.*

It is every small boy's pride that he can make fountains with his own urethra, and urination plays a big rôle in the ritual ceremonies of primitive peoples. Urination has always a fascination for the small child—his own urination and that of animals and of other people.

Play of this kind falls into the same classes as are noted on pages 75–76.

CLASS A

R.D., Boy, aged 5½. While he was playing with water the rubber dog got water inside it, and this delighted him. As he squirted it out, he said excitedly, "Oh, he's tiddlin'; that's fine, look, he's tiddlin' "; and soon after this he tried to fill the rubber doll with water, but the hole was in the back of its head. He turned it upside down, dragged its legs apart, pointed to the part where the penis should be, and laughed.

P.T., Boy, aged 4½. Worker gave him rubber dogs with a hole under the body. He soon discovered he could fill them with water and squeeze it out. This caused much delight and pleasurable excitement. It was obviously associated to urinating for some time, because he exclaimed, as if rather naughty, "I'm making the dog wee-wee." This was repeated in excitement. Then he went on to the rubber syringe, and filled the dogs with this. He sometimes caught the water from the dogs in the bath. Rubber tubing was also filled, and he liked to see the water coming out the other end, but was more interested in the dogs than the rubber syringe.

K.T., Boy, aged 9. The dolls were then bathed, head and all. Water was poured into the rubber squirting doll and K.T. said he kept it in him until he went to bed and then he let it out all over the bed. He also let some out walking—or, if hit on the head, he turned round and squirted water.

Many children give a name to the act of urination such as "tinkling", suggested by the sound, and show a very evident interest in this noise.

CLASS B

Imaginary reproduction, in act or in symbolic creation, of excretory organs.

A.T., Boy, aged 8½. He used rubber tubing as a hose, directing water over his hand and round the sink with evident satisfaction. He asked for the squirt, and showed keen delight over this, the contents being aimed at a hole above the tap on the balcony. He held the squirt in front of his penis and tried to see how far away the water would go.

On another occasion. Playing with a rubber tube, he first used it for washing the tank out, then, holding it at pubic level, directed it up as a fountain, altering its direction and form by squeezing the tube. He was entirely engrossed and pleased with this for some time, staring fixedly at the wall (through the fountain) and at the same time plucking at his knicker opening.

On another occasion. His water play, when alternately squeezing and relaxing rubber tube, and making powerful spurts of water, was very similar to urination.

P.T., Boy, aged 4. He turned to water, placed a large rubber tube on the tap, and turned the tap well on, and for some time watched the water gushing forth, sometimes in stream, sometimes in fountain. During this play he was in an emotional state which almost reached that of complete satisfaction. This play appeared to be associated with power in urination. He smiled contentedly. He held the pipe lower and as near the position for urination as possible, saying, "Yes, it all comes out of Peter." He discussed his father and brother in this respect, and said that his brother could only make a small trickle.

B.C., Girl, aged 7. Her attention was at first held only by articles which could be filled with water and then emptied, or the water squirted out. She then found the rubber tube, and, holding it at the level of her bladder, made the tube shoot water upwards, saying she was making fountains.

Class C

If children are allowed space, material, and opportunity to follow out their interior themes to what seems to the child logical conclusions, play of one kind which develops one theme will pass, by connections that are clear in the child's mind, to another theme analogous to it, and continue in this new element to develop the old theme. A vivid example of this development of interest is the intimate connection that so often appears in free play between urination plays, bathing, and the eternal fascination of water.

Play with water takes an infinitude of forms.

Water in itself is delightful. For example, take the play of:

E.H., Boy, aged 4½. He asked if he could play with water. The rubber tube was put on to the tap, and he had great pleasure in trying to grasp the "ribbon" of water as it flowed from the tap. Then he tried to squeeze the tube, and it was pointed out to him that he could control the flow either by squeezing the tube or turning off the tap. He seemed very pleased, and asked worker to put the stopper into the sink, saying he wanted to sail some boats. He was very particular to have one big boat and two small ones. He also picked up a small iron boat which sank. He tried several times to float it, finally putting it upon the big boat, which was at once over-balanced. He picked up a model wash-basin with tank and tap and got great enjoyment from running water through the tap, and again tried to catch the stream of water.

On another occasion. He chuckled with joy when the water splashed over, and laughed aloud when he discovered how the stream was diverted when he put his hand into it. He jumped up and down with delight, saying, " Now you do it." He repeated this a number of times, taking turns. He splashed himself until he was soaked, but refused to protect his clothes either with a pinafore or towel. Then he held up his face to be wiped, saying " My face is all wet ", beaming at worker.

In this example can be seen the sheer sensuous joy that the qualities of water in themselves produce in children. Together with this goes the excitement of " discovery " that takes so large a part in evoking childish and, for that matter, much also of adult delight. Every child has the experience of producing water from within its own body and finding that this can be controlled by itself, given out, withheld, and in boys the force and direction of the stream directly influenced. From this and the experiene of defæcation the idea of filling and emptying is very vivid to the small child. He feels himself full, then empty; his bladder full, bowels full, stomach full, and then all these three either voluntarily or involuntarily emptied. Pouring, filling, emptying, and filling again plays a large part in the natural occupations of children, and by these actions they seem to make intelligible to themselves the physiological processes they experience.

The following extracts from the Institute notes illustrate play of this sort:

E.H., Boy, aged 3½. He wanted the water toys, and we went through the form of my asking him to put on an overall and his refusing and suggesting I should play with the water. He talked the whole time, and towards the end of the afternoon fell into a curious sound like a pleasurable moan, which he kept up through everything he did. He filled and emptied vessels, one into another; not very full, but continuously. He had sand on one side and water on the other, and put handfuls of sand into the pots of water and poured water on to the sand-heap. He gave the rubber dog and child a bath. He added jugs, pots, watering-cans, animals, boats, motor-car, to a large basin which became half full of water, sand, and objects, and he continued to fill each new thing with sand and water, and between whiles to bang sand into a mould and turn it out.

R.L., Boy, aged 6½. He came into the playroom and went from one thing to another tentatively, then, suddenly, made a bee-line for the water room. He looked round, then he turned back to fetch a chair to stand on. He turned on the taps and enjoyed the rush of water. He filled a big jug with water, overfilling it. He then took cups and filled and emptied them, and tossed the water up on to the wall with great enjoyment, banged things about and flung them down—the long boat, the cups, the jug, etc. Many things for no apparent reason he called " Dirty thing "—a cup, a pastry roller that bobbed up in the jug, etc. This roller he then flung across the room.

On another occasion. He went straight to the water. He asked for all the squirting toys. I gave him them all. " Is that all? " he asked. Then he squirted for a little. I had then to put in all the toys, the ducks, fish, everything, including the boats—the sink was crowded out. Next he turned his attention to the pumps, bath, basin, and lavatory, and played happily with these, pumping, filling tanks, and turning on taps.

C.S., Girl, aged 7. She became interested in little by-play with water and then in the water. She turned the tap, poured water through the tube, and was delighted with a rubber doll that squirted through a hole in its chest. Then she began to splash water about, and, taking bowls of water to the window, she then squirted it over the balcony and the leads. After that she got a broom and more water and, with cries of delight, swept the balcony, making the water drip into the yard below.

B.C., Girl, aged 8. She played at filling the toy lavatory, showing special interest in the emptying mechanism. She held the lavatory over a bath and this over a jug, so that each emptied itself into the vessel below it. She held the bath patiently, although her fingers got stiff, until it had completely emptied itself. She then filled the sink through a rubber tube and floated boats, fish, and a crab in it. She removed all but a celluloid boat, which she threw from a distance, making a splash. She then emptied the sink, remarking on the funny noise the water made running out. She said it was like thunder.

F.S., Girl, aged 10. She remarked upon the three lavatories with pleasure, but showed equal interest in the fish and ducks. One doll was seated upon the lavatory. She remarked that the other doll was straight and could not sit, so she put it in the bath. She filled both lavatory and baths with water with the squirt. She seemed to enjoy the squeezing action of the squirt, and was very intent upon filling the large duck with water through a break in its side. She showed delight when she tipped the duck and all the water rushed out. This action appeared very important to her, for, hearing another worker say that she was ready for her when we had finished, she murmured that she *must* fill the duck. She then filled it full and emptied it out, then stood straight up, threw up her head, and sighed. This movement seemed to express a certain amount of satisfaction and of achievement, but most of all relief at having accomplished some task or enterprise.

It will be noticed that a certain aggressive element appears in several of these examples. Aggression is a natural accompaniment of urinary experience in a normal "masculine" boy. He wants to "p" farther than his little friends, to push out his urinary stream with greater force than he did last time, to display himself in so doing—to strut, as it were, like a cock, and crow over his achievement. All this comes to expression in water play. Examples:

E.H., Boy, aged 4. He was delighted when he saw all the water toys. He filled the sink with water and put in all the boats. As the sink was rather high, he stood on a chair, and worker passed him what he wanted. He pushed the boats about and seemed uncertain whether he preferred the large ones to the small ones. Then he took them out and asked for the "quack-quacks". He put them in and made two of them "fight", and one he pushed under water and said it "drowned itself". He found the baths and wash-basins, and worker showed him how to work them, and he spent a long time filling baths.

Girls enjoy using substitutes for the organs they lack.

J.D., Girl, aged 6½. She went to use the water squirt, and this seemed to satisfy her. She became calmer, and enjoyed filling the squirt and aiming chiefly at the top of a head (made with plasticine) and at its ears. She also squirted water with the syringe down into a tray, then up at the face, down at the tray and up at the face in a kind of rhythm.

F.V., Girl, aged 7. She abandoned the "world" for water, and began to be violent, splashing water over and flinging the toys about. The ones she did not want she hurled from her. She seized other children's toys, in spite of protest, and began squirting water down people's necks, etc., until Dr. Lowenfeld took the squirt. She was annoyed, and only accepted the situation because the squirt was actually in Dr. Lowenfeld's pocket.

P.T., Boy, aged 4. Rubber figures were squeezed with great force when filling them, and squashed right under the water: not only the filling but the crushing and drowning mechanism were evidently of importance to the child.

B.G., Boy, aged 9. He squirted water from a very high level into a sand tray. A wooden boat already there was swamped. An Indian was selected from the world cabinet and pelted with a stream of water until he and the boat were overturned, and the tray flooded. Dry sand was mixed with the wet, and a glorious mess ensued. He plunged his hands into it with evident satisfaction, but when asked what it felt like he said, "Oh, it's rotten."

R.D., Boy, aged 5½. While playing with water he put a policeman in the jar and drowned him. The fish, etc., were added and called "mixed pickles". He returned to a dog, calling it "baby boy", filled it repeatedly with water, and then squeezed it flat. Then he hammered it with his fist, saying, "I'll kill him. I'll kill him." Then he tried torture, trying to put the dog's paw through the mangle. He then put its tail through and said it was dead. Then it was drowned.

Without a very large number of examples it is impossible to give any idea of the richness and variety of children's play with water and the number of interests that such play can express or symbolise. There are so many properties about water that are an endless fascination to a child. It is to some extent mouldable; that is, it can fill things and be emptied out again; it can be clean, dirty, or coloured; it can make other things clean or dirty; it comes out of apertures with force; it can be used to "drown" things and to knock things over. Moreover, upon water boats can float, toy divers can sink and be "drowned" and "come to life" again, fish can swim in it and ducks upon it, and it can be swilled over floors.

From one of the characteristics of water, that of pouring, comes children's delight in the pouring of other substances. Mrs. Isaacs[31] provides this example:

"*12.10.25.* In the sand-pit, Tommy put some sand up the leg of his trousers, and let it fall down again, saying, 'See how it pours.'"

The following are notes from a case seen in private:

Girl, aged 7½. She went to sand tray and was delighted to find that adding water to dry sand made it possible to mould the sand into solid forms. She ran backwards and forwards with great energy between the sand tray and the taps, being particularly amused in trying to direct the stream of water from a long rubber tube attached to the pipe into a jug. When she had filled the jug, she dashed to the sand tray and emptied it on to the sand. It was impossible to convince her that the limit of the sand's capacity to hold water had already been reached, and she continued to pour water on the sand tray until the larger half of the sand had disappeared. The idea then struck her that it would be nice to have dry sand to put in the water, and, after experimenting for a little while with a shovel, her face lit up and she took the same jug as she had used for the water and began filling it with dry sand, and poured it out on the water in the tray. She pointed out to me as a great discovery that pouring with sand was just like pouring with water, and as the water had made little bubbles in the sand, so the sand made little conical heaps in the water. When the larger part of the sand was soaked up, she entered on the next phase of play by putting her hands backwards and forwards in the sodden sand, testing the feel of it, patting it and stroking it, and carrying out quite elaborate experiments with the making of channels in the sand down which the water ran. She was not satisfied until she had tried everything she could think of with engineering feats with sand and water.

3. *Plays concerned with defæcation*

Children of all ages delight in defæcation plays, either directly transposed to toys, as in the case of the child Jane, quoted on page 74, or in symbolic by-play of their own experience; and the same interest persists in many people in the form of excretory jokes, into adult life (see p. 8). With children, defæcation play is very often combined with interest in bathing. As with urinatory and mouth plays, defæcation play also falls into Classes A and B.

CLASS A

E.H., Boy, aged 3½. He washed a celluloid doll in water and sand, and fetched a boat, more dolls, a lavatory, a bath, etc. He explained the mechanism of the lavatory to worker, and later seated a doll on it and pulled the plug, then knocked it off the seat. Later he admired the dressed doll, but rejected her because her clothes would not come off and so would get wet, and chose a small china doll instead, which he directed worker to undress. He seated her in the bath with water, then sand. Later this doll was also made to " sit down " and pushed off roughly.

P.T., Boy, aged 4. The two toy lavatories and their workings thrilled him, and he was most intelligent with these, and at once grasped their working and then liked to pump one into the other. The celluloid doll and the bath with pump also pleased him greatly. Then suddenly, with a half-questioning, half-enquiring look, he placed the doll on the lavatory seat and then, as if I had done it, not he, questioned, " What is he doing? " I replied, quite unmoved, which I think surprised him, " Oh, either No. 1 or No. 2, or whatever you call it." After putting the doll back in the bath, he did it again, and said, " What is he doing now? " I said, " Well, he has had his bath, and now he is doing No. 1 before he goes to bed, just like you do."

I.D., Girl, aged 4½. She put dolls in baths and washed them, and also seated them on the w.c. quite naturally, saying, " You'd better go to the lav now." Then she played pouring.

Stanley Hall also gives similar examples in *Aspects of Child Life and Education*[13]:

" F., 3. Her dolly often wants to go to the water-closet, and is tenderly put on the stool by her little mother.
" F., 6. Beats and almost breaks her doll because she ' wets herself most every day.' "

CLASS B

Play of this kind is rarer among children, but does occur. It is difficult here to give examples, as the play consists of gestures and fleeting expressions, and these are hardly ever observed sufficiently in detail to be recorded. But in films, and particularly some American films, and occasionally in movie animal cartoons, can be found abundant evidence of this interest, and a derived interest in the parts of the body allied to defæcation.

CLASS C

Just as urination play becomes inextricably associated with water play, so the fact of defæcation leads inevitably to ideas concerning the products of defæcation, and the opinions of grown-ups about them.

The addition of water to sand inevitably suggests the bodily product that is so like this in appearance, and the connection between the two substances is quite clear to small children. Extracts from Institute records show this:

E.K., Girl, aged 8. She made a mound of sand, wetted it, planted a small cage at the top, and put "me" in it, buried up to the waist. Nothing else was in sight, and I was to die of hunger and thirst. There was also an imaginary serpent, in the hole, that bit my feet. Large wild aminals were next put on the mound, all converging on me, and trees in between. Then "E.K." was planted walking up the hill to save me. She knew the magic word, which was "Quig-quig Kaka-re-kiki" and this kept the animals at bay. There was great joy over "kaka". ("Kaka" had for long been her name for fæces.) All the mounds were "kaka", and I was "deep in kaka". She pointed to herself and said, "Kaka comes out of here", and then flung herself on my knee laughing.

M.M., Boy, aged 2½. Another boy had been playing with sand and had left it very sloppy in one corner. M.M. had watched him with interest, and, as soon as he had gone, he went to the tray and began stirring up the wet sand. A jug was full of sand, and he scooped it out and dropped it in spoonfuls into the set sand and squashed it flat. He did this with great interest, and, when asked, said it was called "Bum-bum".

R.D., Boy, aged 6. He made pies with damp sand, calling them Christmas puddings, after having built the sand up into a pile in the middle and patted it down with a spoon. He said during this that he meant to be a farmer and to grow flowers. He would also keep every kind of animal. Worker asked what he was expecting most at Christmas, and he said, "To smack your bottom." He was hitting the puddings with a spoon at the time and pretended to smack worker.

Susan Isaacs[31] reports similar forms of play:

"*18.6.25.* Tommy and Christopher spent half an hour making what they called a 'bee-wee-pie' with sand and water. In the sand-pit, in the morning, Paul and Harold, and, later, Frank and Dan, had 'made try'—mixing sand and water with their hands—'with salt', they said. Frank piled it up on a brick in a loaf shape, and Paul called it a 'loaf of try-bread'. Harold did the same, and said, 'When someone wants to eat a try-loaf, we'll give them this.' Paul and Harold went on with this 'try-bread' for some time, and said they were going to cook it. Harold later asked Mrs. I. if she would like a loaf, and took her some."

Out of an extension of this interest comes a child's interest in and love of "dirt"—mess and materials that are mouldable. All children pass through a stage of intense interest in moulding, crushing, and dirt, if the opportunity for the exercise of it is presented to them. But such opportunity by no means always occurs, since the messiness of small children is an aspect of their life that most easily and early comes under adult disapproval. In many children this ban becomes effective enough to be incorporated in their own estimate of themselves, and to prevent a display of such interests even where the opportunity occurs. In such children it is often possible to see the action of both impulses at the same time—the primary interest itself and the ban that condemns it. Such examples as the following from the Institute records illustrate this situation:

P.T., Boy, aged 4½. He had a tray full of very wet sand, which he pushed about and piled with a slate, damming up muddy ponds and then letting them rush out. He leaned his arms in the tray and got them muddy to the elbow, and showed them—a little pleased and a little shocked, and glad to have them wiped. He began slopping the mud on to the floor with great satisfaction, and when there was an extra plop he murmured, "Da."

B.R., Girl, aged 11. The utensils were messy., so we took them to the sink to wash. She picked the least messy. There was a porridge-like mess in the bowl. She appropriated this and said it was clotted cream, then poured it and stirred it. She enjoyed the mess another child had made and put the dough on worker, but was very careful not to mess her own fingers, and only by proxy to enjoy the cheeky things that the other child did.

On another occasion. She accepted dough obediently, saying she was quite interested in cooking. She is not in a high enough class to learn it at school, but mother lets her help and is going to teach her to cook properly. While talking, she mixed flour and water with a spoon, taking care not to get it too wet. Then she began kneading. She got tremendous satisfaction from squeezing the dough, but this was quickly counter-balanced by the dislike of feeling her fingers messy. Later she enjoyed painting the dough to make "jam tarts".

Other children respond to this ban not by adoption but with resentment, and, where disapproval has been severe, tend later, in the face of opportunity, to explode into violent exploitation of these sensations. Examples:

B.D., Boy, aged 9. He came in his overall, saying, " I am very dirty, oh, I am so dirty ", and went straight to the pudding-basin in which he had mixed a mess last time. The top had got dry and hard but the inside was still squashy. He began to make an incredibly repulsive mess with water, dough, and sand, and the stuff in the bowl. He sloshed it about in the tank, mixing it with water, mopping it up with a rag, and putting it back again in the bowl, and showing great delight and enjoyment.

M.B., Girl, aged 12. She noticed wet sand tray into which she threw her painting-water, then plunged her hands in, saying it was "ever so cold, but felt lovely "; she kept drawing them up and down the tray for quite a while with keen enjoyment. She patted the sand so that it became even messier than before, and said it reminded her of the sea.

On another occasion. She turned her attention to a fairly moist sand tray. Worker piled up sand, at which M.B. threw handfuls, trying to hit worker's hand before it could be withdrawn. Her enjoyment in the messy nature of this occupation was very keen.

The facts about defæcation that are of most interest to a very small child are the emergence of this substance from an aperture and its having been moulded into particular shapes. Another attractive quality is that the continuity of this substance can be broken at different points by the action of the child himself when he makes use of his anal sphincter. Both a mincing machine and a grinder are in action similar to this quality of the child's own body, and in the Institute playroom the mincer and grinder are among the most popular of the play apparatus. For example:

E.H., Boy, aged 3½. While looking for a train, he found the grinder. He put "cakes " left by another child into it. He was very interested in seeing this dough and plasticine "coming out ".

R.L., Boy, aged 6½. He was putting the mincer on the shelf, but stopped to put plasticine through it. He asked for yellow plasticine, and a piece of old yellow was given to him. He put it through the mincer, and was pleased when he saw it coming through looking different.

J.J., Girl, aged 7. She found the sausage-meat grinder. She complained that the plasticine did not come out fast enough. She squeezed lots of plasticine into this machine, and wanted to squeeze much more. Eventually she took a really large lump of plasticine and made a cake of it.

B.R., Girl, aged 10. She made models of Squeak and Wilfred in plasticine. Then she passed on to mincing plasticine, which afforded her much satisfaction. For about ten minutes no plasticine came through, but she continued to grind and grind, in hope that it would appear. She said, " I love mincing." Finally it came through in several long pieces. She likened it to bananas, and then rissoles such as her mother made.

Sometimes grinding and water play go together. For example:

E.H., Boy, aged 3. He was putting the powder from grinding from one small tin into a larger one. He emptied the tin on to the floor and then began filling the tin from the pile. Suddenly he asked for water. He then fetched the doll's teapot and filled it at the sink, then watered the pile on the floor and also the grinding machine. Then he fetched a water-cart and filled this repeatedly from the teapot, showing great interest in its tap. Finally he emptied the water out and went to the sink. There he filled the teapot and emptied it into a jug. When this was full, it was emptied into a basin, and this was tipped into the sink and the whole process repeated. Water coming out of the spout of the teapot while water was running in especially interested him, as did the bubbles. He turned the tap on harder and harder, finally letting the water run into the basin with much splashing, to his evident pleasure.

We have already spoken of aggression in connection with the idea of urination. It is inevitable, as a moment's thought will show, that, by a parallel extension of ideas, ideas of aggression should arise also in connection with defæcation play.

Children emotionally regard the mouth and the anus in much the same way. The breaking-off of the stool in the act of defæcation is similar to the act of biting. Both these actions are violent and destructive, and if they were carried out on other objects and in real life would tend to inflict pain. Hammering, piercing, and cutting up soft and mouldable substances, and their use as missiles, express extensions of these ideas.

Examples:

E.H., Boy, aged 4. After seeing plasticine alone in the cupboard and rejecting it, his attention was caught by the grinder. Seizing it and plasticine, he worked with great energy, and worker was ordered to hold her hand under to catch the bits, which were each time put back and ground again. The largest lump was finally put on top (it was much too large to go in). Later it was taken out and put on the table to be hammered with a crescendo of violence, the hammer being held above his head and smashed down as hard as he could. Each time he did this, he said, " That would hurt, wouldn't it? " (A statement rather than a question.) A nail was driven into the lump until it became quite hidden. Each time the plasticine was hammered flat he deliberately dented it and made holes with a hammer, viciously jabbing rather than hitting.

N.T., Girl, aged 2½. She pretended a brick was a head and grated it through the mincer on to the floor. The she cut it up. She asked if worker wanted a baby, and, if so, worker should take it out of the cupboard. Worker did so, and then she started to feed worker's doll with pieces she cut from the head.

G.P., Girl, aged 3. Plasticine gave her great pleasure. Her little fingers were too weak to manipulate or cut it, so worker gave her two tins and a wooden mallet. She placed the tin and hammered it down, then tore away the plasticine and dug out the piece which remained inside the tin. This was done many times until the tins were hammered too flat to use. She also hammered and otherwise destroyed several figures which worker made for her.

B.R., Girl, aged 10. She took a mallet and hammered plasticine into pancakes. Worker helped to make pancakes and sausages for Dr. O. B.R. cut plasticine with scissors and gloated over the sensation. She became increasingly insulting to worker, smashing her work, remarking on her personal appearance, throwing plasticine at her, and pushing it inside her clothes. Then she played peep-bo round a screen, under the table, many times, then mounted the table, and pelted worker persistently and vigorously with plasticine.

Charlotte Bühler has called attention to the primary nature of the child's experience of negative or hostile emotion. This is expressed in play in a number of ways, and a large variety of examples of aggressive action in play will be found scattered throughout the chapters of this book. This aggression is sometimes expressed directly and sometimes by symbol, and occasionally is directed against specific parts of the body of a plantasy object. Here are instances:

D.F., Boy, aged 4. He could use only his left hand, as the right was bandaged. He delighted in cutting off heads, arms, legs, etc., of plasticine figures, and also hammering them, or pulling the heads off and throwing them away. The throwing away seemed to cause the greatest satisfaction. Finally he could not wait until the figures were complete, but seized them from the worker before they had arms or legs.

J.D., Girl, aged 5. When taken into a room by herself, she rode on the rocking-horse and I left her to come at her leisure, whereupon she gave a series of raps in order to attract my attention. Eventually coming to my table, she picked up a pair of scissors and proceeded to chop off the heads, legs, and arms of plasticine figures I had made.

B.G., Boy, aged 10. While playing with water and a rubber doll, he took both its hands and made it smack its own face, and then he hit it in the face. Then he made it smack its face again. When the worker asked why, B.G. replied, "Because I tell it to." It had a tiny hole in the nose, and he looked through it and another hole in its head at the worker. He then squirted water through it, and eventually bit off its nose, leaving a larger hole, and threw it down.

The same ideas can be expressed in other ways; for example:

M.M., Boy, aged 2½. There was a pram beside him and he tried to poke out the doll's eyes with scissors. Then he tried to cut the eyelashes and the nose, and tried again to poke the eyes with his fingers. He found a small brush, and dabbed it in the water and on to the doll's face, hair, and bedclothes. He did this several times, and later on in the afternoon he made another attempt to dig the scissors into the doll's eyes.

R.D., Boy, aged 6. He began experimenting with water in a teapot and a funnel on either end of the rubber tubing. He then placed a rubber doll head downwards in a jar, crammed it in, filled the jar with water to drown her, saying that her name was "Dirty Snob". Then he went to the sand tray and washed sand through a large tube, also a toy man which he found inside. He then made a large sand-heap and placed a glass jar, filled with soldiers and sand, upside down and buried it. He fetched water and poured it over to drown them. The sand was then washed off the jar, the jar reversed and reburied, and a flag stuck on top of the mound.

On another occasion. He poured sand through the holes of a Meccano toy. Then he threw sand in the air and also directly on the floor. He pelted the paper on the wall with sand. Plasticine nose and eyes were put for him to throw at. He threw at them till he got them off, then became very excited, throwing sand all over the wall. He agreed to sweep it up and grew quieter. He asked for the squirt and squirted the walls and people, a plasticine face on the wall being squirted only once, though he agreed it looked like worker. He also squirted water down a tube.

A child's first year or year and a half of life, besides containing many and varied digestive and excretory experiences, provides for him manifold experiences of the senses. Since there not much else to occupy his attention, a young child's sense experience is particularly acute.

Children in a free atmosphere show keen interest in touch sensations, and greatly enjoy experiments with tactile feeling. The following are examples from the Institute records:

A.T., Boy, aged 9½. He piled sand on to one side of the sand tray and **sieved** it on to the other. Worker was told to put her hand on the tray, and this was covered gradually with sieved sand. She was then told to move her fingers first under the sand, and then come out gradually—the fingers first. He moved his own hands backwards and forwards through the sand, and made the worker feel the difference between the sand and the stones. He then picked up handfuls of sand and let it trickle through his fingers; then he let it fall from a height with a flop. The stones were taken off the tray and he spread the sand out over the whole tray and said, "It is finished."

B.R., Girl, aged 11. When mixing dough, she first made it too wet, and then added flour. She said, "Isn't it a lovely feel?" and then, "Do you like making pastry?" after which she used a rolling-pin.

D.S., Girl, aged 13. For a short time at the end of the afternoon I gave her the pastry-board, rolling-pin, flour, and water. She made dough, then proceeded to squeeze and mould and squeeze. Her eyes glowed with pleasure. She could not get on to using the rolling-pin and making pastry for sheer joy of handling it. She threw a ball of dough into the air, catching it with a firm grasp and pleasure. "It's a lovely feel," she said. "You try and see what it feels like." She handed it to worker, who agreed. She was then called away. Excitement was sustained throughout.

M.B., Girl, aged 12. Seeing the dry sand, she said she would make a desert and flopped into a chair. She took pleasure in sifting sand through her fingers, remarking that it felt "just lovely". She also enjoyed squeezing it.

I.D., Girl, aged 4. She filled an india-rubber dog with water, which she squirted out with some pleasure. She then asked for sand and made a mound, which she said was a castle. She put some toy money into it and enjoyed burying her hand deep in the sand, remarking, "It does feel nice."

M.B., Girl, aged 8. She plunged her hands into sand and churned it about, exclaiming delightedly at the feel of it, "I love messy things." She wanted to make caves and tunnels, but the sand was too wet, so she transferred some of it in the sieve to another tray. Finding the sieve made a pudding-shaped mould, she made several of these before returning to her own tray. Mixing some sand with the remaining wet sand in the tray, she made an island in the middle with a narrow strip joining it to the edge. Then she fetched water to make the sea. She put her sandy hands up towards worker's face, touched her cheek with one finger, laughing at the result. She asked to be allowed to wash her hands, and said, "Look, the sand makes your hands clean."

B.D., Boy, aged 5. He went first to the dry sand tray, enjoyed the feel of the sand, picked up a handful and let it trickle back into the tray. He said he wanted water, and moved across to the wet sand tray. At first he disliked the wetness of the sand, and added some dry sand, after which he appeared to feel happier. He commented on his dirty hands with disgust.

Touch sensations allied with moulding interest give rise to pleasure in smearing. For example:

P.R., Girl, aged 10. She was disgusted by very wet dough left by another girl, but she was much interested in cooking and in making things look realistic, and made a " pie " and a "jam roll " with success, and was very much pleased with the results. Then she smeared herself with flour and aimed some at worker with great glee, also throwing some at Dr. L.

Smearing can be done with very many substances, but it is usually combined with experiments with colour.

M.M., Boy, aged 2. Someone had left some painting things on the table, and he started painting—using a reddy brown colour. Then he turned the paper over and smeared the other side with a dark bluish colour. He was very much engrossed in this. Then he started tipping the water into another jar, and finally on to the table.

On another occasion. He found a piece of blue chalk, which he wetted, and then scribbled over the " shop windows". This called forth constant squeals of laughter.

J.M., Boy, aged 9. He wanted great quantities of flour, and used the sand-shovel to it. He then mixed very messy dough, rolled some of it out a little, and went back to the sticky stage, mixed it with paint powders, and put the resulting mess in a pudding-bowl and tied it down with paper. He was very insistent that this must be left for the next time just where he put it, and that no other child should see it.

F.S., Girl, aged 10. She asked to do painting, and, while worker got her the materials, she put the blocks away. The painting gave her great pleasure, and she was neat and her touch was light. She was very interested when she found that by mixing two colours she could produce a third, and spent some time experimenting.

It is important to remember that a child's reactions to olfactory experience are very different, and even the exact opposite from the reactions of an adult. The smell of dung, of manure, or a manure-heap in a farmyard is definitely pleasurable to many small children, and fæcal smells have not the repellent quality for them that they assume for the rest of us in later life.

Recapitulatory play with smell is comparatively rare, and, for the reasons above stated, it is hard to give opportunities for it, yet it does occur. Susan Isaacs[31] gives an example showing this interest:

"Paul said to Mrs. I., 'I hope you smell—you smell yourself.' Dan went to the lavatory to make water. Frank was in the cloakroom, and was heard to say to him, 'Dan, you are a ah-ah-ah-ah-ah-bottie—say that, Dan.' Dan did so. Dan told Mrs. I. that Frank was passing fæces."

Stanley Hall[13] also gives an example:

"F., 4. Came into the room and saw a box which had not been opened. Would not go out to play, and as soon as others left the room tried to open the box. Failing to open it, she knelt down and smelled it."

It is interesting that in the Montessori scale of sense training it has also not been found possible to include olfactory material and the same difficulty has been found in the Institute.

The common association of anal products with eating (which is well illustrated in the extracts from Mrs. Isaacs' notes quoted on page 73) persistently crops up in the play of children. It gives rise to a number of curious associations with taste. Recapitulatory play with taste is rare, and the provision of opportunities for it is accompanied by the same difficulties as occur in the case of smell. No apparatus for taste education is, for example, included in the Montessori apparatus, an omission which might be in the interests of future good cookery to remedy.

The following are illustrations of taste experiments from the records of the Institute children:

P.T., Boy, aged 4½. He cut rolls of plasticine into half-inch beads, and threaded these on a steel rod. He offered pieces to worker to eat, and was thrilled to see them bitten and the marks of teeth. "Was it nasty?" he asked.

F.V., Girl, aged 7. Her desire to lick or taste was shown when given Grip-fix to mend a toy. She put the brush at once into her mouth. She asked, "Is it to eat?" Worker: "No, for pasting. It would give you tummy ache." F.V., taking more, "I don't mind."

Experiments with sound form an immensely important part of a child's recapitulatory and experimental life, but consideration of a child's experience along these lines comes under the two headings of language and music, and does not properly belong to this chapter.

About these sense experiments in *Aspects of Child Life and Education*, Stanley Hall[13] says:

"Experiments in touch, taste, and sound become prominent in the second year, and the latter are frequently carried to an extent which proves trying to the nerves of adults. Active experimenting with taste develops somewhat later. According to Mr. Bell's studies, while ability to carry things to the mouth begins in the fourth month, and some tastes are differentiated at this time, and biting develops along with dentition, active experimenting with taste proper begins in the second year. Children from two to four or five years taste everything. One hundred and eighty-two different articles are mentioned in Mr. Bell's list of objects tasted, including plants, hay, straw, sticks, seeds, paste, pork, rubber, soap, tar, dirt, worms, and insects—in fact, anything 'that can be carried to the mouth or the mouth to it,' quite irrespective of any edible qualities in the objects tasted. Another phase of curiosity in regard to taste is the 'teasing to taste', which, according to the same authority, reaches its height between the ages of seven and ten. One hundred and twenty-two different articles are mentioned in Mr. Bell's list, the majority of them edibles in some stage of preparation, but uncooked mixtures and medicines of disagreeable flavour also figure largely in the enumeration. Experimenting with mixtures of both foods and drinks is most frequent between the ages of five and ten, and a year or so later comes the stage of adolescent testing, when the desire to try everything new in a bill of fare, to sample new combinations and flavours, appears to be a characteristic of the developmental period.

Another aspect of a child's interest in his mouth experiences with which we have dealt is the connection of the mouth with the strange properties of air. There are many ways in which air is interesting and exciting to children. Air will make bubbles in liquids of all sorts; it can be made to produce the tenuous loveliness of a soap-bubble, and strange noises when blown into pipes; but best of all are the odd noises produced by the human body.

A little girl of 3, talking to her brother of 4½, said one day, "Jimmie, if we didn't have moufs, us could talk with our bottoms." "No, stupid," said Jimmie, "we couldn't. We can only make pops with our bottoms." (Privately contributed.)

The following are extracts from the Institute's records showing children's interest in air.

J.B., Boy, aged 7. He enormously enjoyed a game played with a worker of putting water in one end of a tube and blowing through the other, sometimes both blowing together. Sometimes he would hide before the spurt of water came.

B.G., Boy, aged 10. When blowing up a punch-ball, he blew at the fire, and also at worker's face.

I.C., Girl, aged 9. She copied in drawing two round comic faces, choosing a man with the "bicycle pump" in his mouth and a very long-nosed one. She said that the reason the man was so fat was because of all the air he had pumped into himself; it would not have anywhere to get out. She then spoke of a man she and a friend had seen doing the same thing as this man—pumping himself up with a bicycle pump—and said that he was fat already and her friend said she thought he would burst. She could not think why he was doing it, but she was quite sure he was pumping air into himself.

Part of the charm of wind instruments to a child is the discovery that so simple an action as blowing out of one's mouth produces, when done into an instrument, a musical sound.

A.M., Boy, aged 12. He took a mouth-organ and sat down on the arm of an easy-chair, facing the fire. Another boy wanted to "learn playing the mouth-organ." A.M. said that he "just plays" and never tried to play songs. He just knows that there is a different sound in inhaling and exhaling. He and the other boy then tried to imitate each other, i.e. one playing a little tune and the other trying to repeat it, but this was not very exact.

G.T., Boy, aged 6. He started with the tin whistle, and asked me how to produce different sounds. I made him blow, and covered and opened one hole alternately. Then he himself made up a tune with two holes.

Closely linked to the joy of air is the fascination of fire. Air will blow soapy water into soap-bubbles; it will also blow fire into sparks and make the lovely glow of red-hot coals. Fire comes continually into the minds of small children, but only when there are a garden and leaves for a bonfire, or very special arrangements inside a room, can opportunities be given for safe experimentation with it. For example:

A.J., Boy, aged 6. He asked if worker had any matches, as he wanted to make a bonfire, and showed keen delight in the fire when it was lit, shouting to everyone to come and look at his fire. But he would not strike the matches himself. He watered his fire to put it out, then piled on more refuse and then more water, and eventually dug a hole to bury the remains of the bonfire.

On another occasion. He asked for matches before he went out, and on his way to the garden said that it wasn't a very warm day and that a fire would be nice to get warm by. He jumped for joy at the first real blaze, and once, when he had found dry wood and it burnt well, he said, "Aren't I a good boy?" He lighted branches and held them up burning. The match had to be put inside a paper bag to light it, and he also put a a lighted stick inside it. His second fire was made inside the dust-bin, and once he put the gramophone horn on top and used it as a chimney. Coal was fetched from the cellar, A.J. remarking that "his dad had coal too." He was delighted with the idea of sawing wood for the fire, and this and the burning of it occupied almost the whole afternoon. Matches were often lighted for the sake of lighting them, though worker usually had to do it in the end, as A.J. was a little afraid and dropped them.

B.I., Boy, aged 9½. He came in and went straight over to a desk in the room and began looking for a box of matches. He found them and lit several, blowing them out one after the other, and looked round for something which he could burn. He decided that he wanted to burn a "town", and told me to make one for him. I suggested that it should be made in the sand tray, and proceeded as rapidly as possible to make dummy houses, and we both decided that it would be wiser to move the tray near to the tank where the water was. He helped build and with the sand made a seaside beach, putting in four boats and a boathouse. He insisted that all the houses should be placed very close together and at some distance from the sea, and set down people amongst the houses, being very anxious that the people should also be burnt. He then set fire to the town with one match, and fed the resulting flames with everything available that he could find, making a really big blaze. This he then drowned with water from the taps above, and, while pretending to be annoyed, was actually genuinely relieved to discover that only a few of the people were burnt. He then mixed up the burnt papers and the sand with the water, and made an incredible mess, and, having done this, he lost interest in it.

Finally, in our study of those elements of an infant's experience to which attention is rarely directed, we come to the infant's peculiar relation to and interest in the question of holes, or, to put it another way, in the spatial relations of solid objects and cavities.

A child's first experience is that of gaining both nourishment and acute pleasure from the insertion into its mouth of a solid rod-like object, and he reproduces this pleasure later by the sucking of his own fingers. Similarly he becomes early aware of the two other orifices through which substances come, one of these, in a boy, associated also with an occasionally rod-like object.

Though it may be unexpected at first sight, careful thought will show that symbolic reproduction in play of situations concerning rods and cavities must be a natural and even inevitable response in the young child's mind to such experiences, and all educators are agreed that this is so with all children.

If play is to be the medium, as is our contention, for the arguments which a child conducts with himself concerning his experience, it is obvious that this part of his experience must have a place in it too.

In order to provide material for this type of "argument", the playroom at the Institute is furnished with many forms of apparatus in which rods fitting into holes form a part. It is true, as is agreed by all schools of early education, that play with the fitting in and out of such rods and holes is a natural stage in the progressive learning of control of material and the development of the understanding of spatial relationships; but partly also it offers the re-creation of experience which had, at the time it occurred, and so continues to have in a part of the child's mind, strong emotional colouring.

Let us call these two aspects the functional and the emotional use of such apparatus.

EXAMPLES SHOWING THE FUNCTIONAL USE
(I.C.P. RECORDS)

N.T., Girl, aged 2. She pointed to rings and holes, and worker gave them to her. She spent the rest of the afternoon putting on and taking off the rings. She tried the diamond rods and holes, but preferred the rings. She took the rings off and put them on a chair—she did not like to put one ring on top of another—then she put them back again. If a ring stuck, she indicated to worker that she wanted it taken off, and as it was tugged off she drew herself up in a tense movement.

On another occasion. She took out the rods, holding four or five in her hand at once. Then worker put a rod in a hole. She looked at it and started putting hers in holes. She soon discovered there was a right and a wrong end; and carefully looked at each rod before she put it in the right way up.

F.H., Girl, aged 2½. Saying, "I want hammer and nails", she took large nails and put them in holes in the wood. Then she took a large hammer and used it on small nails and pieces of wood, hardly looking at what she was doing.

On another occasion. She took a small stick and hammered it into a hole so that nothing was showing on the surface. When a row was hammered through, she started again at the other end, hammering them back.

M.M., Boy, aged 4. He settled down to rods and holes very happily. First he used the rings, and tried to pile them up, and then he took the diamonds. He kept putting them into piles without the rod, and whenever he had a large pile he chuckled with delight. He put a piece of chalk through one of the holes.

P.T., Boy, aged 4. He was playing with Matador. He hammered and showed great joy in seeing sticks come through the other side, and in pulling them through with pincers. He played with this for a long time.

EXAMPLES SHOWING THE EMOTIONAL USE
(I.C.P. RECORDS)

M.M., Boy, aged 4. Two children were throwing skittles about. M.M. picked up two. "Daddy, two daddy." He put them to his mouth, showed them to his mother, and put one through wire netting and hammered it with the other. Worker made him a plasticine man, with which he was very pleased. He held it tightly in his hand while he followed his sister round the garden.

On another occasion. He found the rod belonging to the doll's cradle and poked it through the letter-box in the "shop", then pushed it right through. He fastened the door shut, and from the outside peeped into the shop through the letter-box. This delighted him, and he played this for several minutes.

On another occasion. He arrived in the playroom with a hollow brass rod and a small celluloid chicken. The chicken was dropped through the rod and fell into the water. Worker pretended that she could not find the chicken. He hid it behind a tray and was full of glee at worker's unsuccessful search.

The ideas behind this type of play can also be carried out with plasticine.

K.T., Boy, aged 8. He took a large lump of plasticine and stuck it on wood and drilled a hole through it. It stuck, and he made a wall round it at which he showed pleasure and pride. Burying the lump of plasticine in the sand, he made a solid heap. Then he made a hole in the top into which he stuck a small round stick, grinned, and pulled it out. He took a great of trouble making a wall round this, reinforcing it with wood.

E.C., Boy, aged 4. He seized plasticine and at once began to make holes, and then a tunnel with a sort of cowl on top. He said, "That is a *Hole*" (great emphasis on the word "hole"). It is a dark place where ladies go. Gentlemen go too, and ladies, and they are frightened and they like it."

Sand and earth can also be used to similar ends.

J.B., Boy, aged 7. Not satisfied with staying indoors, he bolted out into the garden, where his time was chiefly occupied in digging a hole and sticking a long pipe end up in it. He climbed this, and then filled the big hole with water and messed about with mud.

R.A., Girl, aged 4. On arrival she started playing with moist sand, patting it and then making a house. Mounds of sand were then built and holes made in them with a clay stick and her fingers.

G.W., Girl, aged 12½. While playing with the sand tray, she picked out all the animals and noticed the holes on their undersides. She then found a small piece of plasticine and made a tortoise, asking how many legs it had. She spoke of seeing the tortoise swallowed in an earthquake in a hole in the ground. She insisted that worker's plasticine model was better than hers, but was reassured that hers was better. She referred to the holes in the animals. Worker: "We all have holes." G.W.: "Not you—you are different."

Another version of this play is the planting of a very tall stick in the garden and then hitting it down, and other games with long sticks or rods. For example:

T.D., Boy, aged 7. He picked up an iron rod and stuck it up in the ground and then hit the ground with it. He then fetched wooden posts from the house and stuck two in one of another boy's holes. He fetched water, and first poured it into the hole, and then over the posts from the top, saying they were soldiers and were being drowned. Two other posts were then added. He attached a cord to one of these with the idea of making a clothes-line. He was very proud of them when they were made.

R.D., Boy, aged 6. He planted a long wooden stick in the garden and seemed disappointed that it was not taller. Then he hit it with the shovel. He cut the grass with the shears, and then, looking up at the mothers' room, made a disparaging remark about his mother, and shouted to try to attract her, but almost immediately afterwards said he hoped she would not see him. He then planted a tree in the garden.

The same idea is often played out with fantastic colouring in play with tunnels and trains that go in and out, cars that go in and out of garages, and other similar games.

T.L., Boy, aged 9. The toy garage and car continue to absorb his attention. Again and again he seems to be setting himself a difficult, but not impossible task, namely getting a large car in and out of the garage.

On another occasion. He brought a long racing car with him, which he said would be very difficult to get in and out of the garage. He achieved his feat with much care and patience, then announced that the driver was "Laura Cromwell".

P.T., Boy, aged 4. He played with another boy with a large aluminium airship and large bricks. They built a garage and ran the airship up and down the room and into it.

A.J., Boy, aged 7. He played with an engine and bricks, and was very pleased with multiple bridges. He said that the "puffer" must go under all of them, and showed great joy when a successful arrangement made this possible. A "dark tunnel" (enclosed shed) was then made, and the "puffer" must end its journey in this. Big arches were destroyed in order to get sufficient material for it; it was very important to him that there must be no chink of light inside. The engine was bricked up inside completely, but before he left the ends were opened again.

P.S., Girl, aged 4. She asked for bricks and built up quite a good model of an engine and coaches running through a long tunnel.

If the variety of the forms of experience that we have been considering in this chapter be passed in review, it is clear that the writer of the extract that heads this chapter was not far wrong when he estimated the amount that the small child needs to learn (and therefore has to pass through in experience) as exceeding that necessary for a university graduate.

In considering the relation of the child to this mass of material, a very profound fact of human experience has to be taken into account. Experience in itself benefits the human psyche nothing. Experience has to be assimilated and understood before it has any moulding effect upon the personality. Every man or woman of experience knows of many fellows of their kind to whom almost all the events that are accounted significant in human life have happened, who have been through flood, famine, and pestilence, childbirth, marriage, and bereavement, and who have remained nevertheless curiously untouched by them. To affect a human spirit, experience must in some sense be externalised, and, when externalised, meditated upon and re-assimilated into the psyche, or the psyche remains untouched. Play of the nature we have been considering in this chapter, performs these functions for the experiences of the first year of life.

A child who has passed through two years of life has already accumulated a large store of experience. But this experience is totally at variance with all the subsequent course of his life. Nothing after the first year of life is the same as during that year.

What is the child to do with these experiences? Consideration of this point brings another law of the working of the human mind into play. No mind can profit by facts or assimilate statements that are entirely unrelated to similar facts of which the mind is already aware. A fact or an experience to be of profit must be capable of relation in intimate sequence to facts or experiences already incorporated in the mind. Much of the teaching that is often given to the three-year-old is totally unrelated to anything that has previously absorbed his interest. He, therefore, either learns it as a parrot or it entirely passes him by. We have seen the nature of the interests that the child's mind spontaneously seeks for itself. Given material with which to work out these interests, a child will explore his experience with deep and absorbed concentration, and, in this exploration, with skilled and sympathetic adult help, will find his way to understanding and assimilating his experience, and so be ready to absorb the next stage of life's lessons. Failing such opportunities, unassimilated experience clogs the highways of the mind and the child turns a dull and bored eye upon freshly proffered education, having already too much in his pouch of memory that is undigested.

Nor is it easy to exaggerate seriously the importance of these first years of life. Future physical experience is based upon the experience of the earliest years. Failure to understand and assimilate infantile experience leads only too often to failure to assimilate and understand adolescent experience, and this failure in its turn leads to the stunting and malformation of the whole of the rest of life.

It is a common practice to undervaluate the intellectual equipment of young children. Their materials for thought differ so fundamentally from those of the adult that their most serious thought passes too often for failure to think at all. Given opportunity and the proper means, children will carry out processes of logical deduction and investigation that would do credit to the mind of an adolescent. Perhaps this can be best illustrated by an extract from the notes of a child of four, seen in private consultation:

Girl, aged 4. She was playing with a sand tray. She looked thoughtfully at the sand and then at the water and, as if guessing a relationship between the two, she left the sand tray to take a large bowl. This she three parts filled with water and put it on the broad edge of the low sink. Then she began taking spoonfuls of dry sand and thoughtfully emptying them into the water. She looked carefully at the fact that the sand first made the water " dirty ", and then, as it settled to the bottom of the bowl, became darker in colour than the dry sand. She went on putting sand into the water, but was not able entirely to soak up the water in the bowl. She then poured the contents of the bowl away and took some dry sand, a largish heap, which she put on the bottom of the sink and then very carefully sprinkled water upon it with the rubber tube, noting and pointing out to me that addition of water to sand in this way not only brought about a change of colour in the sand, but that the water disappeared altogether into the sand. At this point it was time for her to go, but she gave litte moans of dissatisfaction, and insisted upon taking instead another bowl and putting a very little water in it. Then, by taking the partially wet sand, she was able entirely to mop up the water. Having succeeded in doing this, she took another bowl with this time a very little water indeed, put a large shovelful of dry sand in it, and not only soaked up all the water, but left the sand with some of it not turned into the dark brown of wetness. Finally she put it under the tap and washed the whole thing away. Then she gave a deep sigh of satisfaction and went away happy.

Looked at from the surface angle of a small child playing about with water and sand this appears to be a very ordinary hour of play. But if the sequence of events be taken and carefully studied, it will be seen that the mind of this child moves perfectly logically from step to step, assimilating each step as it goes, and building carefully and concretely the following step upon the logical deductions of the first, as is done in all forms of careful and logical thought.

Just as in the meditation and day-dreaming of adults experience of one kind melts insensibly into memory of experience of another kind, and both are combined with phantasy, so, but in a greater confusion, does children's recapitulatory play of one kind merge insensibly into another, going forward, returning upon itself, changing its shape, and interweaving itself with phantasy, so that these examples, chosen as they are to illustrate something of the underlying structure of early play, give an unreal impression of separateness. In the actual play of small and medium-sized children, all varieties in a play afternoon tend to be woven into a single fabric, and that fabric to express the total reaction of the child to its own past experience.

Given freedom to work out this experience and the right kind of aid in its difficulties, a child will pass through the experiences of its early life without becoming over-attached to any of them. Without such opportunities it is only too easy for that stunting of the intellectual and emotional life to take place of which the existence of so many *blasé* adolescents and bored and vindictive adults provide evidence.

CHAPTER V

PLAY AS THE DEMONSTRATION OF PHANTASY

"Play is a very serious matter to the child. To him it is a business which absorbs his whole feeling, thought, and action."

JEAN PAUL RICHTER.

" PHANTASY " is the modern name for "castles in the air", and has found its way into general usage with the coming of knowledge about the deeper and more obscure processes of the human mind. " Phantasy ", as it is generally understood, is the name given to that kind of mental functioning which earlier was called day-dreaming or reverie, and which stands in opposition to imagination and controlled thought. Imagination is a creative activity with a definite relationship to reality; phantasy rules in a world of imagery, controlled entirely by the individual's desires. Phantasy is "the stuff that dreams are made of", and the material out of which, in the early childhood of men and races, many of the conceptions of the outside world are forged.

During the period when it was held that man was ruled by reason, and that therefore the ultimate appeal should be to reason, phantasy was frowned upon as an evil tendency of the mind, an activity unrelated to fact, one to be definitely discouraged as leading to serious ills of mind and character. Modern work in psychology has led to a revision of this conception, and to the discovery that reverie and day-dreaming, phantasy and dreams, are not accidental happenings or bad habits, but are linked with the deepest processes of the human mind.

Every experience leaves some trace upon the total personality, and it is unlikely that any experience, even in infancy, can occur without the accompaniment of some, however rudimentary, intellectual concept of that experience. Even, therefore, in an infant, every emotional experience will be accompanied, however vaguely and crudely, by a mental picture of the nature of that experience. But since the infant has no means of testing theory and reality, and no material for the formation of correct concepts, the picture he makes to himself, however distorted it may be, will appear to him as fact. He will, therefore, be unable to distinguish the making of phantasy from the perception of reality, error from fact.

Not only is this true, but it is also probable that concepts formed in the infant mind build themselves up and bind themselves together by much the same associative laws as operate in the mind of the adult. But how hard it is to gain contact with the mental processes of a child! How far we stand from the smallest understanding of his concepts! Long ago this difficulty was finely stated by Sully[15]:

"Observation of children", he said, "is never merely seeing. . . The phenomena of a child's mental life, even on its physical and visible side, are of so subtle and fugitive a character that only a fine and quick observation is able to cope with them. . .

"Things grow a great deal worse when we try to throw our scientific lasso about the elusive spirit of a child of four or six, and to catch the exact meaning of its swiftly changing movements. . . [Children] feel unskilled in using our cumbrous language; they soon find out that their thoughts are not as ours. . . And how carefully are they wont to hide from our sight their nameless terrors, physical and moral. Much of the deeper childish experience can only reach us, if at all, years after it is over, through the faulty medium of adult memory. . . Child-thought follows its own paths. . . Possibly by and by we shall light on new methods of tapping the childish consciousness."

Writing at about the same date as Freud was beginning his work, it is interesting to note that he continues:

"Patients in a certain stage of the hypnotic trance have returned, it is said, to their childish experiences and feelings. Some people do this, or appear to do this, in their dreams. . . These facts suggest that if we only knew more about the mode of working of the brain we might reinstate a special group of conditions which would secure a re-emergence of childish ideas and sentiments."

We are well served if we take his remarks on play and "imagination" (which we should now call phantasy) as a starting-point for our study of this phase of play in children.

"It is surely to misunderstand the essence of play", said Sully, "to speak of it as a fully conscious process of imitative acting. . . When at play he [the child] is possessed by an idea, and is working this out into visible action . . . We talk, for example, glibly about their play, their make-believe, their illusions; but how much do we really know of their state of mind when they act out a little scene of domestic life, or of the battle-field? . . .

"Such play-like transmutation of the self extends beyond what we are accustomed to call play. One little boy of three and a half years who was fond of playing at the useful business of coal-heaving would carry his coal-heaver's dream through the whole day, and on the particular day devoted to this calling would not only refuse to be addressed by any less worthy name but ask in his prayer to be made a good coal-heaver (instead of the usual 'good boy'). On other days this child lived the life of a robin redbreast, a soldier, and so forth, and bitterly resented his mother's occasional confusion of his personalities."

Piaget[32] has brought forward valuable evidence to show that the child before the age of six or seven is autistic in thinking, centred in himself and content with his own views and conceptions of the world. In his studies of children's answers to a series of questions, he brings very strong evidence to show that these concepts are made, not of perceptions of fact, but of wholly fantastic material.

Before the age of eight or nine, children do not use words to communicate their *ideas*. In many children with a poor grasp of language this handicap continues several years later. Yet long before even the first word is acquired by the infant a network of phantasies has come into being in his mind.

As this network grows it will contain ideas and concepts concerning himself, the outside world, and his relation to the outside world, and the relationship between one part and another of that world. It will be derived from his sensory experience, his thoughts about his sensory experience, his emotions concerning the agents that produce, or appear to produce, that experience, and the figures, animate and inanimate, that populate his world. It will be a three-dimensional phantasy in which feeling, experience, imagination, and memory cross and recross each other, layer interweaving with layer, and experience with experience. It will be expressible perhaps in pictures, and sometimes in action, but for most children this life of theirs will have little, if any, connection with words.

In older children, pictures derived from lessons, stories, actual or reported happenings to themselves and to other people, are added to this world of three-dimensional concepts, and a structure of words and names for these experiences begins to form itself among them as a matrix for thought.

There is a sense in which very young children are satisfied with this situation, and do not yet feel the strain of unexpressed phantasy. But the dawn of the day on which this strain begins to be felt is inevitable, and at that point the battle between phantasy and concepts of reality begins.

We are concerned in this chapter with play which is the child's method of representing this conflict to himself.*

" We speak well, in prose, only in order to say what we mean," writes

---

*See p. 74 for a note on the child's necessity to externalise his experiences in order to realise and be able to assimilate them.

R. G. Collingwood[33] in a recent book; "the matter is prior to the form. This priority, no doubt, is rather logical than temporal. The matter does not exist as a naked but fully formed thought in our minds before we fit it with a garment of words. It is only in some dark and half-conscious way that we know our thoughts before we come to express them. Yet in that obscure fashion they are already within us; and, rising into full consciousness as we find the words to utter them, it is they that determine the words, not vice versa."

There is a kind of play which performs for children the function which language, according to Collingwood, performs for the adult.

The mental processes of very young children are too inchoate, too unlike the process known to us as thought, to be given definite shape even in phantasy. Play expressions of this state of mind fall for the most part into the forms of play studied in the previous chapter. Such play can occur only when material which is capable of expressing such experience is present.

The next stage to be considered is the change which is brought about by the entry of words into the child's field of consciousness. Words are first perceived by children as names for objects and persons they see and touch, and for actions which they and other people perform. There is at the time they become aware of words, as we have already pointed out, a large mass of conceptual material already in existence in the child's mind. To him this is truth, since he knows no other concepts, and has as yet no means of expression and comparison of his ideas. The new element of words which are accepted by and familiar to his surroundings, now begin to link up with these old and tried concepts of his own.

Stanley Hall[13], in the earlier part of the century, reported an experiment carried out in Berlin in 1869 which well illustrates this process. A Berlin newspaper issued a circular inviting teachers to ask their boys and girls on entering school the meanings of certain words in ordinary use. The result showed the children as being content with meanings to these words which arose from the most superficial contacts of word with word. *Berg* (mountain), for example, stood to all the girls of an upper class grammar school for a neighbouring beerhouse. Lake was something that could have water in it, but where the water might or might not be present.

Stanley Hall later investigated concepts of sight in children, and we have in Una Hunt's autobiography[34] (see Appendix) an invaluable account of the growth of an entirely fantastic connection between an ordinary word (skeleton) and pre-existent phantasies and concepts.

The opposite process also occurs.

Children form concepts concerning external events which are given normal descriptions which bear a superficial similarity to adult meaning, but which imply to the child concepts entirely at variance with those implicitly assumed by the adult. "The sun goes down, the sun comes up—or rises," says the adult, and means the gradual appearance of the sun's disc above the horizon as the mass of the earth's surface rotates. The sun to children "goes down" also, but, as has been brought out by Stanley Hall, to a child it

"*Goes down at night into the ground*, or just behind certain houses, and went across, on, or under the ground to *go up, out of,* or *off the water* in the morning;... or *God pulls it up* higher out of sight. He *takes it into heaven,* and perhaps *puts it to bed,* and even *takes off its clothes* and puts them on in the morning, or again it *lies under the trees* where the angels *mind it.*.. The moon... *follows us about* and has nose and eyes, while it *calls the stars into, under,* or *behind* it at night, and they may be *made of bits of it.* Sometimes the moon is *round a month or two,* then it is a *rim,* or a *piece is cut off,* or it is *half stuck* or *half buttoned into* the sky. The stars may be *sparks from fire engines* or houses... or *God lights them with matches* and *blows them out* or *opens the door* and calls them in the morning."[13] (See also *The Child's Conception of the World,* by J. Piaget.[35])

It is for this reason very difficult indeed to know what is the meaning of words to a child when it uses single words in play. Sometimes the meaning can be deduced from the development of play itself, but more often the play is not sufficiently coherent to allow of this.

Furthermore, children often experiment with words—a word originally meaning one thing becomes spread over a number of other concepts. For example, a visitor comes to stay whose name is Duncan. He is is a nice visitor and invents good games. These games become "Duncanish", and from this strict analogy the word begins to spread, until a wide area of games analogous to those originally played with Mr. Duncan are collected together and christened by his name.

Children have an æsthetic pleasure in the sound of words as sounds; and if a word with a pleasant sound or an amusing association of ideas comes their way, this word comes to be used for its own sake as well as for the whole range of ideas suggested by the associated events. Thus "Duncanish", which struck the children as a nice sound in itself, came in a certain household to be used partly as describing nice things in vague association with the original holder of the name, partly because it was a nice-sounding word, and objects or activities were sought to which this new name could be applied. An extreme form of the same mechanism was the use in a family known to the writer of "going down buttercup lane" as a synonym for defæcation.

Not only is this true, but children often carry over concepts long after the object to which the term is applied has ceased to exist. For example, to a child playing with plasticine, the figure it makes comes alive the moment it has been made, with a life of its own, and this life persists to the child long after all resemblance to a figure has been lost. For example, a quotation from the notes of a private case runs:

A child of three years, after some play with sand, wanted plasticine. I was told to make a man with a very long nose. The man was to be in yellow and the nose in white. Then she said, " I will cut off his nose." This she proceeded to do, and followed it by cutting the whole figure up in small pieces, and as she did this, said " Look, now he's crying [actually at this time there was no " he " remaining]; he doesn't like being cut up." At all stages she referred to him as if he were still present.†

Words being unsuitable to children as vehicles for the expression or realisation of phantasy, therefore, some other medium has to be found, and this medium is play. Children appropriate the materials they find to hand, and invest them with imaginative qualities that make them a vehicle for the concepts, wishes, and phantasies that surge within their heads.

Having created the elements they need for their play they proceed to combine them in ways which enable them to express the underlying ideas they are trying to grasp.

In such play, all the qualities of the elements that go to make up their instruments of expression are inextricably inter-woven; the feel of a jug with the fact that it can hold fluids—the smell and taste of the glue on a wooden toy with its shape. In all cases the more primitive the material the more suitable it is for this kind of use.

An interesting study of the relationship of material to play is found in Charlotte Bühler's paper on *The Child and its Activity with Practical Material* [20]:

> " As to the question *What can one use?* there is a body of evidence collected by H. Hetzer in a research on about 150 children, whose play habits were investigated partly by observation and partly through *questionnaires.* Only one of all these children does not play with home-made toys, and in regard to most of them the mothers are of the opinion that it is better for the children to be without bought toys than without any other of the things usable for play. . . .
>
> " I should like to give some idea of the abundance of material gathered and used by the children. A glance into the long lists of materials used shows:

*Pots	 4	Waste fur	. . .	1
Spoons	 5	Crumpled paper	. .	1
Saucer	 1	*Porcelain cup	. .	1
Comb	 1	Old clockworks	. .	1
Pot lids	 3	*Wooden cup	. .	1

†This is a very common event in children and is very important for the understanding of their ways of thought. To a child, cutting does not in any sense necessarily mean killing, and the person cut up may just as likely come together again. This tendency is well shown in many fairy-tales and myths.

Egg-beaters	2	Briquettes	1
*Bowls	2	Wooden boxes	3
Ironing boards	2	Barrel cover	1
Cleaning box	1	Newspapers	3
Carpet-beaters	2	Catalogue	1
Clothes-pegs	3	Books	1
*Pint pot	1	Envelopes	1
Hand brooms	2	Postcards	1
Brushes	1	Paper	1
*Kitchen measure	1	Playing cards	1
*Cups	1	Old time-tables	1
Sieve	1	*Crock	1
Wash basket	1	Buttons	3
Clothes-line	1	*Old pots	1
Rake	1	Water	6
Watering-cans	2	Stones	5
Baskets	2	Sand	5
Wheelbarrow	1	Sea-shells	3
Hand-cart	3	Sod	1
Carriage	1	Hay	1
Flower-pot	1	Straw	1
Wooden sticks	9	Sheet iron	1
Empty boxes	5	Boards	1
Empty tins	6	Bricks	4
Bobbins	2	Grass	2
Cigar boxes	2	Apples	1
Old paper bags	1	Pears	2
Empty cartridges	1	Pine cones	1
Old bottles	2	*Etc.* "	
Worthless paper-money	1		
Scraps of cloth	1		

If these be classified and analysed, the items occurring more than five times work out as follows:

Boxes	12.	Tins 6 = 18
Stones, etc.		15
Pots		13
Wooden sticks		9
Water		6
Sand		5
Spoons		5

(Stones, etc. = buttons, bobbins, empty cartridges, sea-shells, pine-cones and stones. Pots = all those marked in the original list with *.)

This affords interesting comparisons with the play material given in Chapter II, and brings out vividly the very wide gulf that exists between materials for play (toys) usually chosen by parents and friends for gifts to children, and the material which is selected by children themselves.

Play, therefore, regarded from this aspect, is the fitting of the half-formed concept in the child's mind with a garment, not of words, but of representation.

Such play takes many forms. Let us quote as our first example an incident from Sully's *Studies of Childhood*[15]:

" A charming little master of three years sits at his small table busied for a whole hour in a fanciful game with shells. He has three so-called snake-heads in his domain; a large one and two smaller ones: this means two calves and a cow. In a wee tin dish the little farmer has put all kinds of petals, that is the fodder for his numerous and fine cattle. . . When the play has lasted a while the fodder dish transforms itself into a heavy waggon with hay: the little shells now become little horses and are put to the shafts to pull the terrible load."

And a few pages later he quotes another similar example:

" P. McL., a girl, observed from three and a half to five years of age, was a highly imaginative child, as shown by the power of make-believe in play. The soft india-rubber was to her, on the teacher's suggestion, say, a baby, and on it she would lavish all her tenderness, kissing it, feeding it, washing its face, dressing it in her pinafore, etc. So thorough was her delight in the play that the less imaginative children around her would suspend their play at ' babies ' and watch her with interest. Whilst a most indifferent, restless child at lessons, whenever a story was told she sat motionless and wide-eyed till the close."

In small children the material chosen to express phantasy is always matter that is malleable and has no definite meaning. The phantasies that can be expressed in this way are as shapeless in form as the material in which they are expressed is vague in meaning, and are constructed of many elements. These are examples:

E.C., Boy, aged 4. He was piling wet sand into the circle of an enamel ring, using more and more, and patting it down firmly. Then he made a hole with his finger right down the centre, withdrew it slowly, and looked down the hole, saying slowly, " What a deep, dark hole!"
Worker: " Is there anything at the bottom?"
E.C.: " No!'
Worker: " Would you find anything if you went down the hole?"
E.C.: " Yes, I should find myself at the bottom."
He then emptied the sand out and said it was a pudding.

On another occasion. He walked into the playroom carrying a paper engine he had cut out at home, and went to the dry sand tray, where he made a snake, "a wiggly one", with his finger. He also made two rivers coming from mountains. They met in the middle and formed a pond. Nobody was allowed to swim in it. He continually made circles with his finger in the dry sand, or made circular islands; now and again he buried the palms of both hands in the sand or covered one over with the sand and said with evident joy, "Now I'm the dirtiest boy in the world."

G.D., Boy, aged 6. He went to the sand tray and filled a saucepan with shell-scoops. He then began to fill a money-box with sand through the slot, and noted the comparative softness and warmness of the sand in the money-box. When this was full he tipped it into a mug; when the mug was full the sand was tipped into a boat; and when the boat was full it was to be pulled by a very strong white elephant; and when this was tipped out we should have made sea-sand. (The heap from which the sand was originally dug was not sea-sand.)

M.C., Girl, aged 11. She was playing with sand, and getting her hands very dirty, enjoying making a mess. She looked longingly at this messy sand as if she would like to play with it for longer instead of doing something more definite. When she was told she might, and that she could make mud pies if she liked, she was delighted. Eventually she made two sand shapes with a house on each and some trees on one, and put shells on the bottom of the tray. She said she would like to make a seaside, but as she had never been there she did not know what it was like. Leaving this, she went over to modelling clay, and seemed to enjoy it immensely, but did not make anything with it—only fooled about, making herself as dirty as she could.

In considering this feature of children's lives, we are brought back again to the factor we have noted twice already. In all forms of human life to which we have access so far, there appears to be an impulse to reproduce in some way experiences which have strongly moved the spirit. As far back as we have records of mankind, traces of such expression are found in drawings, pottery, and sculptures, and these productions seem to bear some relationship to the lives and experiences of the people by whom they were produced. Whether these designs are sympathetic magic, e.g. representation of the successful killing of game in order to bring about future success in hunting, or spontaneous expression of delight in past success in, for example, hunting, is an open question, but, whichever version may be true, it is quite certain that there was a connection between the production of these designs and the lives and experiences of the people who made them. Just so is it with children.

Moreover, it is by means of play of this kind that ideas develop. Play is in a sense artistic creation; each piece of play of this kind is a new creation, and its creation is intimately connected with the development of thought, for until a concept has been expressed, or an experience externalised, it cannot give place to another thought.

All the equipment of the playroom at the I.C.P. can be used, and is used from time to time, for the expression of phantasy, but the most significant piece of apparatus is the " world cabinet " (see p. 32) and the sand tray. A child confronted with a " world cabinet " finds material ready to his hand for the expression of almost any sort of phantasy or concept—material that is malleable to his thought, and can give him just the aid he needs in his struggle to externalise his concepts of the world so that he can define them, limit them, and eventually master them.

The advantage of this type of material is that it allows, like a cartoon or a dream, of two layers of meaning:

1. On the surface is the manifest content, the actual scene which is represented.
2. By associative links between the items used to build up the scene, and the child's own past experience or interior life, ideas entirely different from those shown in the manifest content can be expressed.

Children of all ages make use of the " world " material, but perhaps it is more commonly used between the ages of seven and thirteen.

It must, however, always be held in mind, in attempting to follow the lines of thought of a child who demonstrates in this way, that besides the manifest and latent significance, every object used is liable to have three meanings:

1. The obvious one—lamp-post, hippo, rabbit, etc.
2. The correct or incorrect knowledge possessed by the child about the actual animal or object.
3. The significance which the animal itself has for the child. Thus, a rabbit can be an actual rabbit and play its ordinary part in a given scene; it can be a fantastic figure compounded out of fairy-tales, as in *Alice in Wonderland* or Brer Rabbit in *Uncle Remus,* and at the same time it can signify the child's own self, felt as a hunted thing, a thing that would like to burrow into holes and escape.

And not only the " world ", but all the material in the playroom, as also music and acting, can be used to express and work out a child's phantasy problems.

Children use the " world " material in three ways:

1. To display ideas which are quite inchoate to the adult and yet seem to the child to have a logical sequence. For example:

M.B., Girl, aged 9. She made two small caves in the sand. In one she said there was a small animal with some eggs, but a man came and killed the animal, and the eggs were never hatched. She then made a large mound of sand, hollow inside. It was so high that it reached up to the sky, "where Jesus and God are." Up in the sky it was foggy, and the aeroplanes could not see one another. Only aeroplanes could reach the top, and one brought eggs and placed them at the bottom of the hole in the mound, where no one could see them. Some horsemen were placed riding round the mound to keep people away. When the eggs were hatched, robins would come out. Some people wanted to poison the sand, and they emptied bottles of poison about, and in the water, so that children might drink it. People had to be very careful where they took their children, lest they were poisoned. In response to some question about the mound and the eggs, she said a giant had destroyed a lot of them, and wanted to destroy them all, but some were saved and brought to the mound for safety. Across one corner of the tray she built a strong parapet, with a space inside it for children to play in. The entrance was guarded by a soldier, and there was another round the side to prevent people from getting up. The children had to pay a penny to go in, and there were three small children inside. The entrance was eventually closed up. In the distance at intervals there were three men coming to fetch the children home. She called these "fathers". At this point she said several times, "I've finished it now", and wanted to show it to somebody.

K.K., Boy, aged 7. He went to the sand tray and filled a bowl with sand, scooped out the middle, and turned it out on to the tray. He called it a factory. He poked his finger in to make a door, then again from the top, demonstrating the hollowness. Next he put two small cubes on top, as a chimney, and two ladders from opposite sides, which were said to be for the men who were going to mend the chimney, which was broken. Here he took the top cube off, and, after trying it in several places, placed it separately on the top. He fenced his factory round, partly with sand and partly with fences. He added milk-churns, and a lorry to put them in. There was said to be a cherry-tree at the side. He then smashed the factory up and told a story of an Indian man who had come to mend the chimney and had gone through the roof. He made a second building, this time a solid one, saying, "This one won't go wonk!" This had a taller chimney, not broken, and no ladders. Once more he smashed it, exclaiming, "Wonk!" and said he would make a maze. He abandoned his effort at sand walls and made a solid square house. He poked his finger in a number of places on the top—these were windows in the roof—and the house was "a maze of rooms".

M.E., Girl, aged 14. She took a sand tray and got chairs for worker and herself. She made a high central hill and dug a deep moat round it. She wanted boats, two of them; she put one on top, one on the side of the hill. She called for water for the moat and put other boats round in it. Before going home, she put away the boats and flattened and mixed the hill and moat into a slushy Yorkshire-pudding batter, and said she was going to cook it. Worker was her child who had to help her to get the oven ready etc. She would not let worker play with one of her two little friends, but would not tell her why. She was cross and mean to worker, promising to let her go out and then taking her promise back. At last she said she would let worker go and play with Mary, if she would help her by burying her hands and stirring in the slush. She was rather surprised and pleased that worker did so. She went to wash and became a noisy, bully mother again, banging worker and telling her to stand in a corner.

Not only the "world" but drawing also can be used for this type of presentation. For example:

E.R., Boy, aged 13. He chose a purple-coloured chalk with considerable care and drew first a circular contraption, which looked like a basket, but turned afterwards into a turban, an Oriental face, a snake rising out of the turban, and then an appropriate body to the face. All movements were made with remarkable sureness; there was no hesitation whatever, and no pause for thought. The names "Allah", "Budaa", and "Mohomad" were written in, and, on being asked what the drawing was, he said it was a snake-charmer and asked worker to write this title above the drawing. The title he enclosed with a good sweeping line. He reversed the paper and turned an already given blue line, without hesitation or pausing to think, into a minaret type of mosque, and skyline. Without comment he began to draw a small figure below it, and added the words "Vot vot tink" in green underneath, and a curious ellipse in green and blue, and also a spider on a stalk at the side.

Plasticine can serve as well.

A.M., Boy, aged 12. He made grotesques, including an animal with a head at either end. This was changed to one with an immensely long neck which was twisted about for some while, before being made to attack a house he had made. The first onslaught was very diffident and tentative, but gradually more heart was put into the attack, so that the bricks were thrown on the floor with considerable force. The long-necked animal was made to eat grass and said to be suffering from diarrhœa, while mention was also made of it being in a circus. He became decidedly excited at this juncture, making humming noises like an aeroplane while causing the animal to travel through the air.

2. To represent scenes actually observed. These are sometimes literal, when they have the significance of a water-colour sketch, or a drawing done by an adult of a place he tries to remember; but more often the scene is a child's version of its memory, mixed with fantastic additions from its experiences.

Here are illustrations.

J.M., Boy, aged 12. He made a country scene, a field with sheep in a corner, and a farmer going through the gate. A road was made across the middle of the tray, forking, one fork leading to the sea. A horse and cart was driven by a male figure, then a second figure was added 'because he's young; he mustn't be left by himself.' Another cart coming in the opposite direction was driven by a woman. This was changed later to a car which she had won in a competition. There were two houses with gardens, and some men going through the gate of one. The other house was where the woman lived. The farmer's house (a small one chosen, because it was "right in the distance") was placed at the corner farthest away from the field.

M.H., Girl, aged 11. She made a garden, using, most intelligently, mirrors for water; flowers, trees, bushes, and a seat were set out with daintiness and a certain amount of charm. She was very particular that each thing should go exactly where it was put. Another child joined her and they decided to make a hunting scene, and searched with real interest among the drawers for the correct material to do so.

A.B., Boy, aged 12. He wanted a lot of sand. He drew a trench down the middle and then chose two churches, saying he would put them together. Worker suggested that one might be a cathedral. He said it was St. Paul's and the Thames, with the animals in the river. When he had put in churches, animals, bridges, caretakers, house, and dogs and kennels, he said, "That's St. Paul's and London." Firemen and trees were added as an extra. When putting a figure of a priest on the bridge, he said, "That's a monk", and later explained about a dog, "That's a St. Bernard."

B.C., Girl, aged 7. She went to a sand tray and started to make a mound in the middle. A house was placed on this and another in the near left-hand corner. A path was made to the house on the hill, on which were placed a woman and two children. A seat was put at the side, on which she seated a male figure and two children. He was the father, and another male figure on the other side of the path was also a father. He had three children with him. A number of domestic animals, trees, etc., completed the scene.

A.M., Boy, aged 12. He collected all the wild animals available, the big ones first, then the smaller. He made a river in which were placed four snakes and three alligators. The animals were arranged, apparently without much method, in and about the sand nearest to him. A zebra and a llama were placed behind a hill "so they wouldn't see the river." He said he had passed a place at Cobham (Surrey) where they had llamas. Trees were put here and there because the animals were in the jungle. The horses were wild and ran ever so fast. One had a baby. When the "world" was completed, he searched out all the cats and dogs he could find, and made it rain cats and dogs by dropping a handful on to the tray. He picked up dog and made it jump on to the back of a hippo, who took it for a ride through the air. This was repeated several times, and seemed to give him satisfaction. He made a humming noise like an aeroplane while holding the hippo aloft.

J.D., Boy, aged 7. Having got out on a square table wild and tame animals including a rhinoceros, a monkey, leopards, and crocodiles, he went to the "world cabinet" to make a zoo, and put a large monkey into a cage, a hen into a hutch, a small leopard into a hutch, and a large leopard into a cage (J.D. went to the Zoo yesterday). Wild cats were crowded into cages and called "naughty boys". The cages, etc., were then cleared away, and a stout wall of "house material" was made all round the table to prevent the wild animals from escaping. He put a rabbit on a wall in a corner. He then collected more animals, cleared the table, and went over to sand tray left by another child. Here he put more cages and wild animals. He then found and was fascinated by a quick-firing gun, which he fired at me rapidly and with loud reports, not as if to hurt me, but as a destructive noise, saying it made my head ache. The wild animals then attacked me, striking me in the face. He then went to a table on which carts, people, etc., had been left, and took great pleasure in arranging identical farm carts in a long line headed by a larger wooden cart. He then picked out soldiers and arranged them in a single file, and remarked that they were the Salvation Army. Worker: "Where are they going?" J.D.: "To the hall." Worker: "What are they going to do?" J.D. :"Pray to God." A policeman was then added to the army, but later taken away to regulate the traffic. A farmer went to the policeman and charged a lady with stealing apples. Later the farmer also joined the Salvation Army, as did a porter carrying a suitcase, called by J.D. an "Inspector".

The child in thus reproducing what he has observed in scenes he has seen is obeying fundamentally the same instinct as the landscape artist, and showing similar elements of selection, arrangement, and interpretation. The intimate connection between children's play and art has been frequently commented upon by Schiller, Groos, and Hall. What remains to be discovered is whether, given the opportunity, this impulse would prove to be equally strong in all children, or whether it operates only in some of them. Investigations of the reactions of children to "world" material are being carried out in psychological laboratories other than the I.C.P., and from these in due time may come the answer to this question.

Children express something very definite with this sort of play, but it is phantasy and not reality. For example, it is clear that killing has another meaning than real death, since in general, children playing "killing" feel it necessary that people killed should come to life again. For example:

J.D., Girl, aged 5. She was playing with the "world". An ice-cream man was seated with care on his bicycle. When he fell off, he was said to be dead, and was put in the largest boat, covered with sand, and firmly patted down. Then she said, "He's got to stay buried, and then he'll come alive again and be a big boy."

M.B., Girl, aged 8. She had made an island of sand, but the water gradually soaked into the heap and the island subsided. M.B. then plunged her hand into it, stirring the sand into the water with increasing violence until it began to splash over the edge of the tray. While making this "storm", she told worker that the island was full of people, and that they were all drowned (this was repeated with great gusto). Then, continuing in a sing-song voice, she told a story of how the King had come to the island to see the great storm and had been drowned, and how all the people came alive again and went to his funeral. Much emphasis was put on the coming alive again.

B.G., Boy, aged 6. He went to the "world cabinet" and chose a wet sand tray in preference to a dry one. He then made a procession of wild animals diagonally across the tray, saying they were all going over the hill to be killed. One shooting cowboy was placed facing the procession—he was to kill them all. After a pause for consideration, more men were added on the left. They had to be soldiers, and they were to trap the animals. Great emphasis was laid upon the fact that the animals did not know they were going to be trapped. He filled up that side of the tray with soldiers, so that the animals were completely trapped, and said that they would all be killed. He then said they would not be killed, but would be starved to death, and later, in reply to a question, said that they would be shot dead. Worker asked if they would be really dead or if they would come to life again, and B.G. replied, "Come to life again, of course."

An associated version of this type of phantasy expression is "playing soldiers". A typical example:

B.G., Boy, aged 10. He left the window and went straight to the "world" toys and chose soldiers. He played Red Indians against the British, the latter always referred to as "us". He took a long time arranging them, and was very engrossed. Then he drew a dividing-line down the centre of the tray with a piece of pink chalk (otherwise, except for the trenches and lines, he used his hands). He said it was like parting his hair. (The dividing-line was about three-quarters of an inch deep, down to tray level.) He drew secret trenches up each side for "us" to approach the enemy without being observed. The enemy would think that it was a precipice. Figures were placed in hiding behind the mounds with their faces against the sand. He tried to make a tunnel at the enemy end of the passage. The Indians were placed first without great care, except for those in hiding and the one creeping up. He insisted that the latter was dancing. "We" had the greatest care and were arranged and rearranged for about an hour. Several times worker was asked, "Does that look all right?" and he complained that worker always said, "Yes." "I believe if someone asked you, 'Would you have your neck off?' you would say "Yes.'" Worker: "Do you really think I would?" B.G.: "Yes, you would say it without thinking." While making his "world", he sang most of the time. Also at intervals he talked of football. He tried to divide the sides evenly, but owing to there being more British soldiers, "we" were stronger. He remarked also that "we" were arranged more strongly, and he would arrange the others, so as to give them a fair chance. They were rearranged, and a battle and bombing (throwing chestnuts) ensued, worker acting as the enemy. Just before B.G. had won, he remembered the secret trench, brought a soldier along it and said "He's killed", obviously meaning one of the enemy soldiers, though there was no direct attack. He said it was a good battle and pretty even. Then, "This time we'll have them put out anywhere; we'll both bomb them together." He tossed up with worker as to who should have the first shot, with a lump of plasticine. Worker won, and all were killed.

Children sometimes use drawings instead of the "world".

K.K., Boy, aged 7. He was drawing, and started with sky, sun, moon, saying you did sometimes see both sun and moon in the morning; then he drew the ground and a bird, and next a nest with baby sparrows in it and the mother bird bringing them three worms—the father was the one on the ground also getting a worm. He started to make the father very big wings. Worker remarked how strong he would be, and able to fly well, and he immediately said, "They are not really wings; they are leaves."

Second Drawing. Baby birds in a nest in a tree. A squirrel hiding nuts ready for the winter—a rabbit running to its hole. He said (but did not draw) a man was shooting at the rabbit, but the shot hit a rock (later said to be a molehill). One squirrel got nuts from the tree and dropped them and another squirrel stole them. An owl swooped down after a worm on a leaf. He drew a cock crowing in the corner, having just laid an egg. When worker suggested that it would be the mother bird, the hen, who would lay the egg, and then the cock saw it and crowed, he swiftly changed the conversation.

Here we see a child continuing with the same idea in two drawings. This following out of a similar idea in a consecutive series is by no means rare. It is said that Professor William James, upon being asked one day what was to be the content of his lectures during the coming term, replied that he would be able to say when he had given them. He went on to explain that until he had expressed his ideas in words, he was not himself certain of the form they would take.

This is true of most of us. We do not know our thoughts until we express them, and to argue a proposition out with a friend is, not to convince the friend, but to make our own thought processes intelligible to ourselves. Children find themselves in the same position as adults—they cannot know their thoughts, much less their phantasies, until they have expressed them, and the effort of expresson itself clarifies and defines the thought, and enables the child to develop the tendencies that lie inherent in it. But children labour under the handicap that we have already discussed—that words for this purpose are of no use to them, and that very rarely is any material suitable for " argument " prepared for them. The " world " material serves them as a means of representation, and allows them to carry on freely these discussions with themselves. Play representing an interior discussion may best be called

3. Progressive phantasy. In such play an argument (if we use this word in its literary sense), once stated, develops from day to day, and the child works out in his own terms the phantasies that obsess him. The following are examples:

T.L., Boy, aged 9. He accepted the " world " tray and cabinet, and proceeded to lay out a village with a church, which is said to be a very small place right in the country. He went on to make a farm with horses, cows, pigs, etc., at the opposite end of the tray, which was surrounded by a fence. There was a wood next to this, also fenced off from the village. At this point he described a wood he knew, emphasising its quietness and solitariness. A farmer was placed at the gate some way from the house, while his wife was put on a seat close to it. T.L. made a river between the farm and the village, and said that on one occasion ever so long ago it had overflowed its banks and destroyed a house in the village. The farmer was not afraid of the river, because the fencing kept it off his land. This gentleman was given a little girl and then a little boy, who were both provided with ponies. T.L. was delighted with his " world ", stressing its niceness and that all the animals looked fat and happy.

1st Repetition. The village and farm were continued with the houses again very close together. He described it as more old-fashioned than the last place. The road had hollows in it, which made it very dangerous for motors, but few came this way because it was a " No Thoroughfare ". He paid no further attention to the village after he started the farm. The same people reappeared, but they had moved, because it was quieter in this new village. The farmer had a different wife because the other one and her two children were dead, which was just as well, otherwise he would probably have got rid of her, for she was horrid, grumpy, and useless. The new spouse was younger and had a son, Charles, aged nine, and twin daughters, Daphne and Mary, aged seven. Mary had pet dogs, but Charles had a female kangaroo called Kenny. Once more he was extremely pleased with the farm, and said repeatedly, "There is no bad temper here at all; everybody is happy."

2nd Repetition. He laid out the village precisely as before, and deliberately made a hole in the road so that it was dangerous for cars, but later on said it had been mended and was now safe for them. The farmer had moved away to Scotland because of trouble with the head man of the village. The children played an insignificant rôle, not appearing until nearly the end. Charles was put in Kenny's cage and John, who was younger, replaced Daphne. T.L. suddenly announced that there were never any robberies on this farm, nor in the village, nor within a distance of fifty miles. The other village and farm had been subjected to burglaries, which was one reason for leaving it. He was careful not to overcrowd the farm, but nevertheless kept adding to it. He said that overcrowdedness and loneliness were both horrid. He thought the farmer would be moving again because the village people did not care for society. The farmer and the villagers did not have much to do with each other. This farm was considered even nicer than the previous one, and there was the usual emphasis on the happiness and good temper in it.

3rd Repetition. He repeated the village, but it was smaller and less crowded. He said the head man of the last village was so disagreeable that the lord of the country deposed him, and in this place there was no head man. The farm was also laid out as before. Again the children did not appear until much later, because they were less important than the farmer and his animals. T.L. said rather dramatically that at the last farm a horrid man who hated the farmer and animals had poisoned Kenny. Therefore, Charles had to have another pet, and a zebra was eventually selected, after much fingering of the wild animals, because "it is an unusual pet for a boy to keep." He put two crocodiles in the River Tweed, which flowed on the side of the village furthest from the farm, but the villagers never went near it. He thought the farm looked too bare, but took great pains not to overcrowd it, rearranging some animals which he considered too huddled together. Just before leaving, he added another hedge to a side of the farm already fenced all round, and remarked, "I like that hedge and fences, don't you?" This farm was also nice, and everyone in it happy.

4th Repetition. He returned to his village and farms with some interesting alterations. The road had lamps, was in good condition, but had two " No Thoroughfare" notices, because "people are sure to read one of them, otherwise there will be accidents." The villagers kept a motor-lorry which brought things to the farm, and narrowly avoided accidents. The farm now had a road through it leading to a garage, while the farmer and his wife (the only people actually introduced) now owned a car. They were both inclined to drive carelessly, particularly the farmer. Considerable interest was shown in manoeuvring the car between farm and village.

5th Repetition. The church in to-day's village was placed apart from the other houses, near to the " No Thoroughfare" notice, and motors had to park some distance away from it. The villagers now had two lorries (fitted with drivers). The farm had its usual animals, including Kenny, but once more the original farmer and his wife were the only people. The latter, while driving, showed off and ran into a fence, besides nearly colliding with things whilst journeying to and from the village. The lorry-drivers were very reckless, and eventually they collided with each other, and killed the farmer's wife, who was in the car in the garage. No mention was made this or last time of people being happy.

6th Repetition. The village and farm were practically the same as last time, but there was a stream inside the farm out of which animals drank. The farmer's new wife drove him safely to church, though she almost collided with fences, houses, etc. Then the farmer drove recklessly and at speed while T.L. exclaimed, "There is no need for him to do that, he could easily help it if he chose." After many hazardous drives, the farmer overturned the car in marshy ground and was smothered with his son John. A lorry driver came to the rescue, but only made matters worse by overturning on top of the car. The wife escaped, became owner of the farm and married again. (Presumably, although T.L. did not say so, everyone then lived happily ever after.)

The story already related, in Chapter III, of Kristine acting her play is another example of progressive phantasy, expressed in a different medium. Painting and drawing can be used to the same end. For example:

A.M., Boy, aged 12. He drew a racing motor with a man at the wheel. He took up red chalk to make flames, and exclaimed, " It's on fire, but look the man is not burned." Then he hastily effaced it, and reinforced the flames with yellow chalk.

Repetition. He drew a figure which had enormous ears and what looked like a large bust. He did not know whether it was a man or a woman, and quickly rubbed it out, saying, " Waste of chalk." It had a mouth, but no teeth, and the lower part of his body resembled that of a seal. This was pointed out to A.M. and he seemed amused. The hands were like bird's claws, and the figure had what seemed to be a row of buttons down the front. He next drew a racing car seen from above, and began to mark it with white chalk as his father, who keeps a furniture shop, marks the things in it. This, though called a racing car, was the development of the design used for the ears. Worker remarked that a row of straight vertical lines might be soldiers, and he at once began to give them heads, arms, large ears, and legs. Worker asked if they were by themselves, and he drew a much bigger figure, which also had enormous ears, done in red chalk to represent chilblains. The appearance of the ears was exactly like that of the flaming car in the first drawing. Purple was used for its face, with the remark, "Purple with rage." It was said to be someone in charge of the children (not their father). This picture was rubbed out, and a map of the country showing Southend and the mouth of the Thames was then drawn, followed by another racing car in which a figure was seated driving. He made huge white rings all round the car, working towards the centre and getting smaller, and said, " I wonder what that looks like?"

Or a series of similar scenes may be drawn, as, for example, by a child of five years who more than twelve times drew a house, with two trees, two plants, and a path, varying each time in relation to the house. Each drawing gave her immense satisfaction, and seemed to her to represent something definite—an explanation which was fulfilled when the meaning of the drawings was worked out.

A curious fact about children's use of phantasy materials for games is that they need only the slightest properties to be able to build up what are for them completely solid structures. For instance:

C.K., Girl, aged 13. We took coloured wood sticks, and I showed her how the green could be used for fields, blue for rivers, etc. Then I went away. She set out to build a house, using these bricks—the slenderest façade only. Later two side wings were added, making some kind of a cellar effect in front. At the door were placed a little woman who was said to be going out, and then a dog inside the house. She next took some trees, saying, " These will make it look more real ", and set out a park round the house, with one person seated in it, and another walking towards the house. On the road to the house were placed a well-dressed female figure returning from shopping and a Wall's ice-cream man. (To the child, as she talked, this structure was entirely solid, and she spoke about the people going in and out, and up and downstairs, as if the whole house stood completed before her.) In further illustration of this may be quoted the following drawing by a small girl aged four:

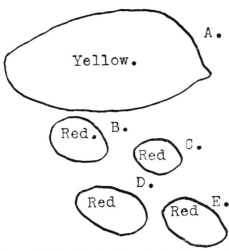

A = body; B and C = back wheels; D and E = front wheels. The child, having drawn this, explained that this was a motor car, and talked vividly about where it was going and the people sitting inside, the whole car being obviously clearly visible to her.*

The same is true with the acted phantasies of dressing up. Much of the charm of the game to the child is the stimulus which is given to the imagination by the absence of the complete uniform of the soldier, or of the robes of the King and Queen; and to press upon a child an elaborately complete acting costume is, in most cases, to rob it of all zest in its game. What has been said by R. G. Collingwood[33] about thought is particularly applicable to children, and to children in this type of play. They do not set out with their thoughts fully developed, awaiting expression, but these thoughts grow as the play develops, out of the interplay between the material and the mind that is working on it. In very few cases does one find a completed synopsis in the mind, which is then expressed in material, but instead that the statement of the first stage of the play (for example, on page 112, " What a deep dark hole ") suggests to the mind the next stage, and it is characteristic of children's phantasy play, if unchecked by an adult observer, that it will move forward simultaneously in several planes of thought at once. Thus verbal association entangles itself with the association of

---

*During the discussion following this lecture a member of the audience quoted an instance of a boy of five who went home and described at great length and vividly how an aeroplane had alighted in the school yard. The only incident that had actually occurred that morning at school was the arrival of the engineer on a motor-cycle. The boys had crowded around this unusual and exciting spectacle.

memory, and this again with the association of selected shapes or of similar ideas; pieces of remembered stories, parts of old games, suggestions from a fellow player, chance resemblances of a piece of material: all are equal grist to the child's mill of phantasy, and only by means of prolonged and minute examination is it possible to discover the concepts that lie behind the phantasy.

Without phantasy play a child's experience remains poor in quality and crude in conception, and it is interesting to note how M. Mead[1], in her study of children in New Guinea, emphasises this fact.

The following are extracts which give some idea of the range and the vividness of children's phantasy play.

E.C., Boy, aged 4. He came into the room as an engine, puffing, and asked immediately for bricks to build a tall, tall, house. " It is not for you and not for me, but for one lot of people, so that they have lots of room to play." (His own house is not very big, but it has a big garden he plays in.) Later he said the brick house was his, and went on to say, " I am not a boy any more, but I am an engine." The house became a yard, with lots of room for the engine to play in. He took a box and made it into a train, running it right across the room, backwards and forwards, to fetch bricks. The train bumped into his house, knocking it partly down, and he said, " I did that on purpose, to see whether there was any water in it; there is not a drop." He then went to an imaginary pump and drew water up from the floor, and took it back, sprinkling it over the house. He started playing with the water tray and its contents, and began making " lemonade " through the toy lavatory. The " lemon " was peeled and put in whole, and the pump cut it up into small bits and it came out " ade". The " ade " gets its colour, he said, from the seat of the lavatory. It goes into the ground yellow and waters the roots and that makes yellow lemons.

On another occasion. He told a lot of stories of how worker was eaten or smashed up by floods, and then put together again by electricity. Finally he said, " Now you cannot be mended any more; you are red blood, and that is much better than you are, because you make things go." Other versions continued for about an hour, worker getting eaten by animals, put into the puddings, going into the sea, and becoming air (" It is nice to be air; I become air sometimes and then I am myself again ").

R.D., Boy, aged 5. Taking chalks and blackboard, he used every colour he could find and drew a house with a very elaborate roof, drawing the roof first. An enormous chimney was added last, with smoke going down to the ground. On worker asking who lived there, he drew two men, one on each side. The first had a very tall hat and occupied one room in the house; the other man had two rooms. They lived apart, having meals separately. The smoke from the house was said to be going in the second man's face.

J.T., Boy, aged 7½. He called the "world" the seaside. It was a mixture of everything, with a small pond in the middle. In the pond were ships, a dog swimming, a goose, and at the edge a crocodile. There were no hedges, fences, or divisions, very few people, and one house. He wanted horses and carts, and fetched two from the mantelpiece. He talked continuously about the different things, and asked if he might have a "second go" and make a zoo. There were a few wild animals available but not many, so he made a farm instead. He wanted to have a rake. Four pigs were put eating at a trough, and he said that was the number in his family (his father, mother, big brother, and Jack). He ploughed a field and sowed seed.

A.T., Boy, aged 9. He made a bed of squared cardboards and called for paste to fix it. He then went on to drawing, asking for a lead pencil. He drew an engine, complete with brakes, whistle, etc., going at a great pace, with the smoke belching from the funnel. Then he drew a steamer, and it, too, was rushing along. Then a cherry-tree, which was very graceful and rather Chinese, crowded with large red cherries, and he drew very rapidly tiny figures in profile, all just alike, scattered about on the branches. He said they were men picking the cherries. He then went to paper on the wall and drew the same cherry-tree, much larger, but this time drawn in separate parts—trunk and each branch, with the same cherries, but no little men.

P.T., Boy, aged 4. He made a ship with blocks, and worker, under direction, made, from plasticine, father, mother, himself, and David, all of whom sailed away, were shipwrecked, rescued, and brought safely home to an elaborate house built for them. The house had a tall chimney, with an external staircase reaching to the top. Father, mother, himself, and David were all put down the chimney and the whole covered over with bricks. They were *not* put down in the fire, but this strange method of entry was adopted for safety. He was methodical in his work, knew exactly what he wanted, and placed his bricks accurately and intelligently. He refused to have more material about than he needed for his purpose.

K.T., Boy, aged 9. A high mound of sand was made and a solid platform (wooden lid of box) placed on it and a square fortress constructed. This was to represent a fortress in the desert. Inside the strong walls was a town. It had four towers, one at each corner and a fifth in the middle of the town. There were two peep-holes in the side of the walls, and one gateway in front with a cannon on top. The gateway was like a tunnel which extended to the middle of the town. Outside the walls there were various animals, one horse, two donkeys, one monkey, and three snakes. There was one man on the steps up to the gateway, and four trumpeters stood in the middle of the town, where they played music. One snake swallowed a baby and completely vanished (in the sand).

On another occasion. Using the sand tray, he made a volcano and bored a hole in the top, at one side. The hole at the side he covered in. " One day the top of the volcano will move and people will discover the secret passage leading to the central chamber, which is full of gold and diamonds." Later he dramatised a flood and drowned three people in it. But the man (the farmer), after everybody thought he was drowned, suddenly popped up again. (His father is a farmer, and he said he is going to be a farmer one day.)

A fascinating problem is the question of the child's own relationship to his phantasy. Children wander back and forth over the borderland between complete identification with their phantasy, conscious make-believe, and a kind of routine play that they know is entirely outside themselves, and yet which is in a way directed from processes within themselves. Occasionally a child is conscious enough of the processes within himself actually to describe them.

E.C., Boy, aged 4. He had in his hand a small toy train of his own, which consisted of two pieces, an engine and a truck. The truck had been broken and he had mended it with plasticine. He stated, " I am an engine-driver to-day, I am not an engine. [Long, deep breath.] You know, sometimes I am my real self, and sometimes I am something quite different from my real self, and then everybody in the house is different, too. Sometimes for hours and hours I am an engine, and then everybody else is an engine, but to-day I am an engine-driver, and mummy is mummy, daddy is daddy, and Wendy is Wendy." This announcement was made with his usual considered solemnity.

Such play, when taken in conjunction with that to be described in the next chapter, in wholesome and normal surroundings, releases a child's energies, in that it makes its own inner life objective, and subject to the moulding power of tangible reality. Moreover, it enables a child to realise the nature of his own preconceived ideas and spontaneous feelings, and by doing so to bring them within reach of comparison with reality.

Minds hold tenaciously to concepts already formed, and to attempt to teach a revision of its concepts to a mind already made up is only to court defeat. Failure to give children opportunity to demonstrate to themselves the concepts they have already made of birth, death, life, and probability, and so to bring these concepts within reach of correction, results only too often in the child's inability later to profit by, or assimilate, even the wisest adult teaching.

CHAPTER VI

PLAY AS REALISATION OF ENVIRONMENT

"The essence of children's play is the acting of a part and the realising of a new situation."

EVERY SMALL CHILD, we have seen, lives in a world of phantasy. Some children sink too far into this world, and tend to withdraw from outer reality to a world within themselves, and so lose contact with reality: but the particular task that every child has to face is to square phantasy with reality.

An infant lying in its mother's arms, receiving immediate attention upon the slightest manifestation of need, cared for in every way by another, appears to us, because it *requires* so much attention, a supreme example of helplessness; but to itself, because it *receives* so much attention, it seems to hold the whole world in its control.

As has been shown in Chapter IV, when an infant meets with frustration, as it must do in the course of the ordinary toilet training of the day, the feelings of rage and revenge which are aroused are expressed in negative movements, and satisfied by aggressive actions and destructive phantasies carried out within his mind.

As soon, however, as he begins to move about and walk, every child comes sharply up against another world, a material world outside himself and which remains obstinately external, refusing to accommodate itself one inch to his desires. Neither screaming nor tears, for example, make any effect upon the table-leg or the closed door. The table remains a table, with its leg and hard edge, whatever he may do about it, and the door a shut door; and, until the child learns the way round that leg, the edge will inflict pain upon him every time he collides with it. Nothing he can do will alter this.

Next, a child's body and himself are not always comfortably at peace. Pains come upon him from nowhere, odd rumblings within that frighten him, and sudden feelings of being sick. Moreover, when the table hits him and the floor comes up and bumps him, and some toy is somewhere where it will not meet his reach and no grown-up is in sight, another strange thing happens to a child: an access of rage invades his person, and for the time being becomes him, and he, the friendly self he knew before, is not anywhere to be found. Feeling like this, he wishes to annihilate his world, as he has wished before when frustrated while lying in his mother's arms. But whereas then his whole world was phantasy, and a phantasy destruction of it was possible, the table and the floor and the toy are now obstinate reality, and to his surprise and chagrin he finds that no intensity of phantasy destruction has any actual effect upon them.

The child, as he approaches the stage when management of himself is forced upon him, thus finds himself, if we consider him as a consciousness, surrounded by four kinds of environment:

1. His own body, his own physical needs and demands, physical appetites and experiences.
2. The material world of objects that surround him.
3. His emotional life; his passions and desires.
4. His family and the other human beings that care for him.

Between the child as a person and this tangled, confused, exciting world into which he has come, there stand, as the bridges between his inner self and it, toys and play, and later, if the school be wise, his work at school.

Every healthy child is excited and interested by his experiences. If he has had freedom for phantasy play, he will have gained much enjoyment and release of energy from it. But this is only half of the picture, for parallel with this enjoyment of phantasy expression of his inner life the healthy child is equally interested in the exploration of the world of fact. Side by side with his pleasure in phantasy, he is engaged in a perpetual endeavour to check up his experience with reality. He wants to understand himself and his world, and to grasp what reality is really like. He wants to see how the people and things that make up his environment *do actually behave*, and, having grasped this, to know *why* they behave as they do.

Out of this desire of his he creates forms of play which are destined both to bring him understanding of the events he sees going on around him, and to give him temporarily some of the glory and the effectiveness of the adults he admires.

The first section of the child's environment, it will be seen, covers not only a child's normal experiences of eating, sleeping, moving, and toilet-training, but also his unusual or abnormal experiences of being sick or being hurt. Stanley Hall and Ellis[13] made a study of children's play with dolls, which shows how all these elements appear in it:

" 90 children fed their dolls with both liquid and solid food; 75 sat at the doll's table; 68 touched food to the doll's lips and then ate it themselves (some speak of chewing it for the doll), or put it in the doll's hand to make believe she ate it; 45 gave it milk (16 of whom imagined water to be milk, and then played nurse the doll in natural way); 36 distinctly imagined the food; 33 set the dolls at table with themselves; 31 imagined or pretended growth, 8 of whom were positive the doll grew, thinking dresses grew short, or pulled doll's legs and found her to measure more; 29 said they never fed dolls or that they couldn't eat; 23 touched food to doll's lips, then threw it away, or put it in doll's mouth and took it out again; 19 distinctly imagined hunger; 19 declared that dolls preferred certain kinds of food to others; 15 were strenuous in urging hunger; 2 said the dolls looked hungry; 9 thought them hungry when they were so themselves; 13 poked food inside the dolls' heads, where sometimes it accumulated and spoiled; 1 broke doll's tooth trying to get food in; 1 broke hole to do so; 12 really put liquid into the doll; 1 had a rubber ball in the back of the doll's head to squirt it out; 13 reported spells of great regularity in feeding; 11, constant regularity; 9 used only liquid food; 7, only solid; 6 imagined they ate without any agency of the child; 7 used empty plates and imagined the food; 6 thought some foods especially disagreed with dolls; 11 seemed to think dolls really starved if not fed; 6 gave foods according to the age; 3 put the food down the neck of the doll's dress; 4 poured liquid food on the front of the dress; 8 always gave the dolls the same food as they had; 1 saw a healthy look in her doll from having slept and eaten well. . .

"Some children put food on the floor near the doll, others think it tries to eat or move the hand toward the food, forgets to eat, prefers cup, bottle, spoon, plate, glass, or to eat with fingers. Some are fed only when children play house, or Sunday mornings, or on coming home from school, or Saturdays, or going to bed, or between meals, or once a day. . .

"Toy cook stoves are a great boon to children during the brewing and cooking age. If children eat too much or prefer the wrong kind of food, dolls are accused of doing the same thing. They are counselled not to eat too fast, nor to be greedy, nor to slobber. . .

"329 papers speak of dolls' sleep. Most of these children are between six and eleven. . .

"F., 15. Nights I undressed my dolls, put on their night clothes, had them say their prayers, and when all were in bed would sing to them."

Not only do the dolls go through all the events of ordinary life, but they are also very often ill.

"In our returns," say Stanley Hall and Ellis, "63 cases of measles, 47 of scarlet fever, 34 of colds, 33 of whooping-cough, 31 of diphtheria, 27 of members injured, 26 of headache, 23 of mumps, 22 of fever, 18 of colic, 11 of croup, 11 of surgical operations, 9 of stomach-ache, 9 of toothache, 9 of leg broken, 8 of grippe, 7 of consumption, 4 of typhoid fever, 4 of leprosy, and 5 were beheaded. The following occurred from two to three times: bronchitis, biliousness, cramp, catarrh, heart trouble, chafed limbs, pneumonia, rheumatism, dyspepsia, brain fever, spells of vomiting. . .

"F., 8. Vaccinated all her dolls, putting in soap.

" F., 12. My baby doll has colic every night, croup, pain, and all sorts of diseases, but the large dolls are very healthy.

" F., 10. Puts her colicky dolls across her knee and they soon recover.

" F., 13. Rubbed red chalk on her doll's face to make a high fever seem more real.

" M., 6. Has dolls that sometimes have three or four diseases at once; they must be rubbed, dosed, the room kept dark and quiet.

" F., 12. Used to give tooth powder for medicine, but stopped when told it would not digest."

Death occurs sometimes in the doll family, and funerals are then carefully carried out, with ultimate burial of the dolls!

" F., 9. Whittled dolls rudely from sticks, buried them, covered the grave with flowers, and in a few days dug them up as mummies."

The vividness of this play to the children is shown in Hall and Ellis's note that " 30 children dug their dolls up after burial to see if they had gone to Heaven or simply to get them back."

Playing out strong emotions which are a subject of recurrent reproof is also an example of this form of play, and many others will be found subsequently throughout the chapters of this book. Stanley Hall notes that

" Quarrelling, talking, answering back, not learning lessons, falling from chair, being ' sassy ', running away from baby doll, slapping baby doll, crying, being jealous, ' won't stand ', ' won't sit proper ', lying, being vain, angry, hitting or falling on small doll, being cross, upsetting things, stealing, flirting, saying, ' I won't ', etc."

are also played out with dolls, and continues:

" 108 children whip, 108 never punish, 80 put to bed, 75 spank, 39 slap, 35 stand in the corner, 34 scold, 21 shake, 20 put in dark closet, 5 throw on floor, 4 broke their dolls, and several hanged them, pulled their ears and hair, stood them on their heads, shut them in a box, threw them up and let them drop, left them out in the cold. The age when punishments are most frequent and severest is below eight.'

Let us now consider the next two sections of a child's environment. Every child as he grows from an infant to a child, and particularly if a second child arrives, finds his early empire slipping from him. He is no longer the centre point of his environment; someone else is now King Baby, and he is forced to accept the second rôle.

The child then begins to feel his helplessnes, his frustration, and a longing to regain his power comes over him. Gradually he sees that understanding of his environment, and of the way one part fits into and affects another, gradually brings him power once more to manipulate this world to his own ends. A study of neurotic children will show how very effectively many children manage to achieve this aim.

Not only does this perpetual drama play itself out in a child's mind, but other forces interweave themselves with the plot continually. Chief among these is the powerful impulse towards imitation. Every child enjoys tremendously playing that he is his elders; having the fun of being, temporarily and imaginatively, in possession of the power of his elders, ordering others about as he is himself ordered here and there, telling them to do things as he is told, without understanding the reason, and making them do things that seem to him stupid. A recent book, *Edward and Marigold*, by Marjorie Thorburn[36], gives a delightful study of the workings of quite ordinary children's minds in relation to this aspect of their environment. Much of the play described in Chapter IV is a child's way of finding himself in relation to section 2 and 3 of his environment: of experimenting with his material world, and of working off his passions and desires upon it. This *motif* continues, but in diminishing ratio, throughout the play years of the child until these three sections cease to be separate parts in his relation to that which is not himself.

Let us now consider section 4. It is a generally accepted psychological rule that it is impossible to understand the meaning of an action unless one can imagine oneself in certain circumstances performing this action oneself. In French justice this mechanism is very seriously employed, and the straightest road to the understanding of the method and motive of a criminal action is taken to be an actual reconstruction of the circumstances of the crime. By a process, then, that may be called empathy, or feeling oneself into a situation through performance of the actions of the actors in the scene, it is hoped to arrive at an understanding of their underlying motives, and the meaning of the actions to those who originally carried them out.

A similar process is very largely used by children. A child observing the behaviour of his family has no means of understanding the meaning of the actions he sees, other than of noting in detail the things his parents, brothers, sisters, servants, and teachers do actually do, and trying to make such links between these isolated facts as seem reasonable to him. He is in the position of a behaviourist, an archæologist, or an anthropologist among a people speaking a language which is unknown to him. He has no guide to the meaning of the actions he sees, and there are very few of them he can spontaneously understand. To grasp them, therefore, the most reasonable course that seems open to him is himself to repeat such parts of them as his memory retains, and make whatever links between them he can.

It is rarely that children give us any reliable indication of the actual processes that go on in their minds, and, apart from the findings of certain psychologists, it is to such books as Una Hunt's biography[34], and certain of the others cited in the Introduction, or to the intuitive perceptions of some novelists, that we must go to gain some understanding of these processes.

To a child, some of the phenomena he observes seem obvious and easy to link together, but some are very perplexing and obscure. In the solution of the problems set him by his surroundings, he is apt to call to his help two aids: the extra knowledge of other children with whom these matters can be discussed, and play of the special "empathic" type we are now considering.

In such a play a child *becomes* mummy or daddy, the woman in the shop round the corner, or teacher, and personifies in himself, item by item, the features of his environment that impress him.

Margaret Drummond[37] shows this process at work in the isolated child, in *Five Years Old or Thereabouts*, as witness the following:

"My four-year-old niece is playing on the floor with her dolls, her bricks, and a dolls' kitchen. We are alone in the room. I am writing at the table, apparently paying no attention. I hear the following:

"'You're a mischievous little thing, putting your legs in my pocket. . . You naughty girl, you're not putting on your clothes.'

"This was repeated many times, with variations, in a singing voice.

"'I think I hear her beating up omelettes in the kitchen; she's not tidying the house. Do you know, auntie, Mary Jane does nothing in our house? She only cooks. She never lays the table or anything. She does nothing. I'll tell you, dear, what I think you should do when I've got you dressed; I think you should go down and tell the cook to tidy the house. I think I'll make the omelettes; and you should sit down and be very quiet till breakfast. She's a naughty girl, she won't dress herself. I tell her a hundred times. Don't you think I'm bringing her up nicely, telling her so often and smacking her too? Everything I tell her just goes in at her left ear and out at her right ear. Auntie's not listening to me and I'm very disappointed. You know, if I don't tie her up tight, she'll go and get cold again the very next day, the very same cold from the very same microbe. I think people are microbes, for they mostly have colds. I wouldn't put on so many breeks as you. You put about a hundred breeks on them and a hundred petticoats. I'm glad I don't dress you the way you dress your dollies, else you'd be crying. Where's her outer clothes? Her dress is here, her dress is here, I've got her dress here. Now, you poor doll. You know my dollies are very unthoughtful for their dollies. They put on a hundred shawls, a hundred petticoats, a hundred breeks . . . crying for heat. . . I'd put you to bed, for you're a naughty girl, I must say. Come on and we'll go downstairs and say that thing to cook. . . Now, you say, "Cook, tidy the house, and mother'll make the omelette."'

"(Squeaky voice) 'Cook, tidy the house, and mother'll make the omelette, and I'll sit very quiet till breakfast. You're not beating that egg right; you're not putting a pinch of salt in it.'

"'Yes, you're a good girl; she's not doing it right. . . Stove in the wrong place. . . Now I'll be cook. It wasn't me that was making the omelette. It was Bridget, Br-r-r-r-idget. Now you make the omelette. Put Bridget away. Put her upstairs in that sack. Now, dollie, get your book . . . keep you quiet. . . I'll get any book for you two monkeys . . . keep you out of mischief, while mumma makes the omelette.'"

Children who have companions in play discover this method of attack on the problem later in life than solitary children, and, once having found it, they make use of it in three separate ways:

(a) They invent games in which they use any object that can be pressed into service to represent features of their daily lives or the life that goes on around them, and the play consists in giving as exact a representation of fact as they can remember or achieve.

(b) They carefully create and enact variations of the actual situation, which embody the fulfilment of secret longings of their own, representing life, not as it is, but as they would like it to be.

(c) They give satisfaction to their feelings by violent distortion of familiar themes in a way that is purely fantastic, and serves to express a hidden grudge or feelings of hostility. This form of play gives expression to the child's concealed feeling about his home, or what he thinks to be the home's feelings about him.

These may be likened to three common attitudes in the creation of literature—Realism, Romance, and Satire.

Let us consider each of these forms of play in turn.

FORM A

This can be carried out in many ways—for example, by use of the "world" and the sand tray. (This way of using the "world" has been touched on already in the last chapter.) In house or "shop" play, or play with a blackboard and benches, or by acting and charades, children often go to fantastic lengths in their endeavour to reproduce exactly the scenes or circumstances they have remembered.

From study of their play a very accurate idea can be gained of the actual atmosphere in a home, an idea, by the nature of things, more accurate than the most skilled social investigation can reveal. Let us consider some examples from Institute records:

G.S., Girl, aged 6. She put on an apron and began to sweep. Then she put dolls in a pram and went out to shop. The older doll was placed at the end, and the baby doll, carefully tended, was put in the best place. The cupboard under the stairs was selected as a shop. She was mother, and worker was auntie who kept the shop. The other doll whined, was scolded and smacked, then kissed and promised sweets. No notice was taken of the baby doll, except to wrap it in silk, chosen for the pleasure of cutting it. During the whole of this play G.S. remained in the cupboard as a kind of base from which she

1. Sold materials to anyone who fetched things from the cupboard.

2. Made a dash to the lavatory to try to get inside with a small boy and his worker (she told worker it was a girl), but the door was locked.

3. Examined the contents of every box in the cupboard. She took the case of soap-bubble pieces, filled it carefully with " sweets " (beans) for her little girl, then mischievously opened the bottom end, scattering the contents. Finally she decided to go " home with her babies " and got back to the playroom.

C.B., Boy, aged 10. He asked if he might go and join the " shop ". A girl was shopkeeper and they had a long and serious buying and selling together in a business-like and friendly spirit. He asked the price, she calculated and weighed, and he paid. He returned to me and laid his foods on the table, naming them with satisfaction, then went back to the " shop " to buy more for the party. Later he went back to the " shop " as shopkeeper and set out a row of silver plates all along the window and set his foods upon them and wrote tickets with their names and prices. It all looked very neat and smart and handsome and appetising.

C.K., Girl, aged 12. She chose to play at school. There were the usual preliminary arrangements of inferior table and chair for pupil, and superior table and chair for teacher. She appointed me as the child, sent me on errands, kept me sitting, etc., whilst she prepared a whole battery of lessons: drill, reading, writing, arithmetic, sewing. But there was no material. She was distinctly harassed and hit me hard with her ruler. I was made to write out " I'm very lazy " fifty times.

E.J., Girl, aged 3½. She played with a doll. It was ill, and the doctor came in and told her to put the doll's feet in water and the stomach-ache would be better. She became ill from eating too many dates which her father had given her.

I.S., Girl, aged 9. She drew houses with the blinds down. Worker asked if it was a funeral. She took no notice, but wrote later, " Preparing for a funeral day." She then drew the funeral, the coffin being labelled " Dear Tom ". The man of the house was 32 and the wife 31, and he had a big boy and girl who gave cushions of flowers. The wife gave a cross, and a brother gave a cushion.

Play of this type is partly purely imitative, and partly arises out of the desire to understand the actions the play represents.

For example, a small child seen in private who was rather backward, and very confused about shops, played as follows:

Girl, aged 5½. She was very keen to play shops, but quite confused about the difference between buying and selling, and wanted to do both at the same time. She set out the "shop" facing her, and I was told to go a long way away, and not to come until she was ready. She then spent considerable time pushing and pulling the drawers and moving things about, but clearly had no idea of what "being ready" meant, and no clear aim, because when she said that she was ready and I returned, there was no coherent arrangement of the things to be sold, or any reason why some were set out and some were not. She insisted that the box of money should be open on the right-hand side, where it chanced to be the first time that we had played the game. She allowed me to take some money to pay with, but was not at all clear as to why I should do this. She has not any idea of money at all.

From then on it became clear that she had watched her mother on her shopping expeditions very carefully, and hoped that by remembering and repeating the actions she had seen they would become intelligible to her. For example, at a certain point she would say, "May I write this down?" and proceed to make motions of writing, like a shopgirl or shopman writing the bill. At one point she asked for a coin and pressed it on the paper. All this with a great air of importance but with no coherence. When I asked for an "apple" or a "cabbage", she found it and very laboriously tried to wrap it up in paper, but it did not seem at all necessary to her that she should give it to me. Sometimes she did, but sometimes she left it beside her and forgot about it. She would accept money from me, but had no idea of giving change, and she had an ineradicable idea that she should also pay me. This arose probably from a confusion of identities in her mind—she wishing to play the rôle of her mother who pays as well as of the shopman who sells—and also from the fact that, having seen a shop attendant come back with money to give to mother or nanny, she thought that the shopman was also paying mummy or nanny.*

Children often repeat the rôles they observe their parents filling. Here are examples:

R.L., Boy, aged 6. He put the boats and ducks in the water, and then started to wash and clean everything, telling me to dry them. I said he was like mummy doing the washing-up. He said, "Yes, and you be my little girl."

---

*During the discussion following this lecture a member of the audience quoted a boy reproducing in play the business of the milkman selling milk to individual customers. He would give no milk without money, and used little bits of paper for money.

He then said, "Pretend to sit on the lavatory", then he came and pulled the plug.

Then he imitated daddy, who is a carpenter:

He sat on a bench and drove nails into a piece of wood, hammering one piece of wood to another and pulling nails out again. He said he was making something, but when another boy asked him what, he did not know. He collected a definite number of tools, sent me for a pencil, and used them all correctly, but without definite end; he made pencil marks on the wood, he sawed, he drove in nails, he pulled them out again with pliers.

E.H., Boy, aged 3½. (He prefers to be mummy rather than daddy, and a woman worker is made into daddy.) He went to the dolls' house and picked up a perambulator and put a small doll in it. Then he picked up the feeding chair and put a baby doll in it. Worker asked him if he were Daddy, and he said, "No, I'm mummy and you are daddy." He repeated this later in the afternoon, telling worker not to forget it. He put a naked doll on a bare bed. Worker suggested that dollie would find it hard and cold; he said "No, it's only wood." He put several vessels, which he first filled with water, on the kitchen stove; one was for tea, another was soup for to-morrow's dinner, and there was something for to-morrow's supper. As each meal came along, he drank the contents of the vessel without offering any to "daddy". Then he took each small vessel, one at a time, and filled it at the bathroom tap and then put it on the fire. He did this with about six small vessels, and at a second tea-time worker was given a cup of tea.

On another occasion. He found a tool-bag and started sawing and hammering, remarking, "Dad says he'll give me tools for Christmas. Dad is a good carpenter, but he won't let me use his saw; he says it's too sharp." He tidied up his own tools. On a later date he sawed, and hammered nails, and pulled nails out. He said his dad had a screwdriver and would not let him use it. He asked several times for a larger saw, saying the one he was using was small.

In playing the parental rôle children are apt to pick up the family's language:

R.D., Boy, aged 6. He was restless until he got to the house game. When asked if he lived at the top of the house, he said, "Yes, and the landlord would bloody well turn us out if he could." I said that putty was used for mending windows and he said, "It takes a long time to mend a window." Worker: "Oh, no, it only takes a few minutes." R.D.: "It's taken the landlord more than two years to mend ours, and he hasn't done it yet."

One girl reproduced a hospital with great care:

I.C., Girl, aged 9. She was the doctor and nurse, and arranged two beds, a table, and two chairs. Worker was told to be the mother and bring her child in a pram, and then wait in a queue. I.C., as the doctor, then received us. She had ruled off paper in columns and asked the name of the child and its complaint. I said I did not know what was the matter with it—it just seemed ill. She said it was influenza (after looking at its mouth), and that it must be an in-patient for three weeks. She put it to bed and got it to sleep, and I was allowed to look at it after it was asleep. No visiting during the three weeks was allowed, for fear of upsetting it.

It is difficult to realise how early in life children learn to observe accurately and to retain pictures in the memory. Here are striking examples:

N.T., Girl, aged 2. She spent a long time with the doll's cradle. She took everything out and then put them all back—not very carefully. Then she took it out again, and, having found two small dolls, she put them on a very small blanket and started to cover them up, but when she found the mattress she changed them on to it and continued covering them up. She put each blanket right over the dolls and then folded it back, so their faces showed. While she was doing this she sat on her tiny chair, and so had to bend forward to reach the dolls on the floor, but always, after fetching something, she sat on the chair before attending to the dolls. Her play was occasionally interrupted by short spells at the dolls' house, where she poured out imaginary cups of tea, and drank them. All the time she was at the dolls' house she had her back to the worker and took no notice of her whatever. Then she saw a basin containing water, also a small kettle, pans, cups, etc., on the table. Immediately she began filling various articles with water and pouring out again. She was particular to empty each vessel completely. This was especially noticeable when emptying the kettle. She was unable to get the last of the water to pass through the spout, but eventually managed by turning the kettle completely upside down.

F.H., Girl, aged 4. She was pleased with the dolls' house and arranged the furniture and dolls. Three good dolls were put to bed, but the naughty one who swore was left in the sitting-room. One was in the kitchen cooking the dinner, and got knocked over rather roughly. The child was pleased. She got two irons out, and spat upon them in a professional manner.

Reproductive play is serious work to the child who creates it, as this example shows:

S.P., Girl, aged 4. With two older girls she was playing the house game. She was attracted by the tiny things, setting them out neatly and laying the table nicely for a meal. When we all sat down to a meal of sausages and bread, she took it very seriously, cutting up her food and drinking the water. Afterwards she helped to wash and dry up and put the things away. The whole thing was intensely real and serious to her, and gave her satisfaction rather than pleasure. She played whatever part in the group was assigned to her as thoroughly as she could, and she did not seem to be acting a part, as the others were.

Stanley Hall's story of the sand pile (in *Aspects of Child Life and Education*[13], pp. 142–56) gives a large-scale example of that sort of play, and a remarkable feature of it is the children's adaptation of their play to the actual circumstances of their town.

Let us turn now to the second form, that of variations of actual situations embodying the fulfilment of secret longings, or a representation of life as the child would like it to be.

Every human being yearns at some time or another for a life different from his own, and children are no exception. Caught as they are within a routine and a set of circumstances that are fixed by their surrounding adults, able to alter only minute portions of their environment, they have, in consequence, no outlet in reality for their half-conscious wishes and desires, and therefore they express these desires in play. It is this aspect of children's play, next to that of group games, perhaps, to which the attention of writers has hitherto chiefly been given.

For instance, in his *Studies of Childhood*, Sully[15] gives the following examples of the lonely child expressing his yearning for a companion in imaginative creation of substitutes:

"When a little over two years old, and for about a year after, 'I had a habit of attributing intelligence not only to all living creatures, the same amount and kind of intelligence that I had myself, but even to stones and manufactured articles. I used to feel how dull it must be for the pebbles in the causeway to be obliged to lie still and only see what was round about. When I walked out with a little basket for putting flowers in, I used sometimes to pick up a pebble or two and carry them on to have a change: then at the farthest point of the walk turn them out, not doubting that they would be pleased to have a new view!'

"A lady friend, a German, tells me that when she was a little girl, a lonely one of course, she invented a kind of *alter ego*, another girl rather older than herself, whom she called 'Krofa'—why she has forgotten. She made a constant playmate of her, and got all her new ideas from her. . .

"Mr. Canton's little heroine took to nursing an invisible 'iccle gaal' (little girl), the image of which she seemed able to project into space."

Later Sully comments:

" I fail to understand what Professor Mark Baldwin means by saying that an only child is wanting in imagination. . . . In his emphasising of the influence of imagination and external suggestion the writer seems to have overlooked the rather obvious fact that childish imagination in its intenser and more energetic forms means a detachment from the sensible world, and that lonely children are particularly imaginative just because of the absence of engaging activities in the real world."

For many children, and for most children at certain times, some feature of their environment presses too hardly upon them, and the way out that is left to them is the re-creation in play of the same environment, but with the painful features remodelled to their heart's desire.

To be satisfying, play of this kind must be realistic. It is rare, therefore, to find children expressing this kind of play by means of the "world". More usually a child chooses as his instruments the dolls' house, the dolls' pram and bed; or in another mood invents plays about house and school in which he and other children take part. The child identifies the object absolutely with the imaginative part it is to play, and is deeply hurt by adult failure to realise its nature. Sully again gives a good example of this characteristic:

" When . . . he was just over two years old L. began to speak of a favourite wooden horse (Dobbin) as if it were a real living creature. ' No tarpenter (carpenter) made Dobbin,' he would say; ' he is not wooden but kin (skin) and bones, and Dod (God) made him.' If anyone said ' it ' in speaking of the horse, his wrath was instantly aroused, and he would shout indignantly: ' It! You mutt'ent tay "it", you mut tay *he*.' He imagined the horse was possessed of every virtue, and it was strange to see what an influence this creature of his own imagination exercised over him. If there was anything L. particularly wished not to do, his mother had only to say: ' Dobbin would like you to do this,' and it was done without a murmur."

The following are some examples from the I.C.P.:

E.C., Girl, aged 9. (Daughter of a street hawker and a laundress.) Choosing the " shop ", she gave worker all the available money and set to work in a businesslike fashion putting sand into bags for sale. After a time she said that she had a little girl called " Catty ", who was nine years old. She went to school, but also helped in the shop, which was called " Daphne's ", but this was said rather indistinctly and might have been " Catty's ". They did not live in the shop, but with father in another house. " Catty " had to go somewhere with her father that evening. The shop closed at 8, but she had to stay where she was until 5 o'clock. (To the child of a street hawker a shop seems paradise.)

I.S., Girl, aged 10. (An unwanted step-child with no sisters, coming from a very poor home.) She started on the house game in a very businesslike manner. The children were left to sleep while she, as "Mrs. Jones", attended to the laundry and other household tasks. The biggest doll was the youngest child. There were three, Eileen, Fred, and Rose. I.S. was deeply absorbed in the game.

On another occasion. Two china dolls were put in first the "private" bath and then the "public" bath together. The main theme of her play, twice repeated, was a poor person's house next door to a rich man's house. The poor house was overcrowded. In the rich house, which was large and had a garden, there were few children. The owner was a policeman. Gradually the garden and house of the poor were enlarged and all the nicest things were given to them. The rich people were said to "show off", and were given a peacock and a dog which was not a good watch-dog.

D.S., Girl, aged 12. (A city child who had once stayed on a farm and liked it very much.) She was making bedroom furniture with coloured bricks. She says she hasn't a nice bedroom of her own; she shares it with her sister. Later she started to make a world, but could not tell one much about it, only that it was a farm with a road running through. She used three small bridges for seats with people on them. She said she had stayed on a farm and she liked looking after the chickens. Butter was made once a week. She made a small hill for the sheep, and put chickens and other animals about the farm. Worker suggested that she should draw thhe farm, and she did a bird's-eye view of it, on the whole very accurate.

A.J., Girl, aged 6. (The second of two children who does not get on with her brother and who lives in a slum.) She and worker were playing being at home. She sat me beside the fire with mosaics to play with, and a baby in a cradle. She tidied the dolls' house and played a little with the mosaics, and then we went out to the park with baby, taking toys for me to play with. We ate food in the park. A.J. brought seven jugs and basins of water, which represented tea, coffee, etc., which she drank and wanted me to share. We came back home and went to bed and shut the door, and I then woke up to find Christmas presents waiting. (Her actual mother is harsh and unfriendly, with a tendency to meanness.) Later she put me by the fire, with baby in a cot, while she made plasticine cake. In the middle of cooking she battered the wall savagely with a rolling-pin. She meant to make four cakes, but grew tired after making one, and I was told to make the others. Then we each made a highly decorated one. We put them on the "stove" to cook. She then brought in four bowls of water, which she placed on the table. I had breakfast and went to school. She was a nice kind mother.

On another occasion. I was made to wheel the baby round and round the room while she made pies with wet sand. I had to say, " I am going to see auntie. Hooray, nobody knows." Then we had a party, and we ate pies and drank the water. I was then put to bed and Christmas presents were brought to me ready for next morning. One of the presents was a tall baby chair.

On another occasion. She decided the floor of the playroom needed to be washed. This she did very thoroughly, washing every corner of it and moving all movable furniture. She also washed the tables and every corner of every shelf of the cupboard, standing on the table to do the top shelves. If she couldn't quite reach a corner, she would say, " Will you do that for me, please?" She looked up once, saying, " I am mother." Another time, " I am a real mother now." Her mother does not let her wash the floor.

M.E., Girl, aged 14. (Second of two children, the other being a boy. Owing to the father's desertion, she has been farmed out nearly all her life with various relatives.) She played house. Worker was mother; she and another girl were the children. Mother sent the children out shopping. They returned with the things, and were sent out again, returning with other goods as the shop was sold out of the article ordered. Mother went out, telling the children to be good, and she returned to find them reading, so went out again. When she came back a third time all the chocolates but one had gone. M.E. told a story of how an old beggar woman came, and, while M.E. was getting her something, she stole the chocolates. The children were smacked and sent to bed, and mother went to a party. The children got up and bought some apples (with money their uncle had given them), and gave them to their mother, who forgave them and sent them out to play. While they were out, they threw stones at the greengrocer's shop and broke a window. The greengrocer came and complained. Mother smacked the children and sent them to bed. They cried and said it wasn't them. Later mother came up to see them, but could not wake them, so sent for the doctor. He said they were dead; they had died of broken hearts from crying so much. Mother put them in the dust-bin. Someone then came to say that mother was to go to prison for treating children so badly. The children were found to be alive, and were given a new mother, but they soon started crying and wanted the real mother back again.

In plays of school, the obvious re-creation of the situation which suggests itself to a child is that of the reversal of teacher and child rôles. This re-staging of the situation shows certain standard varieties.

1. The child as the teacher, with every detail carried out meticulously:

C.B., Boy, aged 9. He asked to be allowed to play school. He was the master; a girl and two workers were pupils. He played the rôle well, and actually worked out the sums to see that they were correct. He told us to write about *Treasure Island*. He threatened to hit us on both hands twice and also on the bottom, repeated it, and then said, "Twice on both hands, not on the bottom." He left the girl as mistress and went off to write reports. He called me "Joan" and the other worker "May". He said my work had been poor (which was true) and "May's" good. I said I did not want to take it home to show my parents, and he said then he would give it to them.

I.S., Girl, aged 10. She played school with a younger girl and worker. She had her turn as teacher and then it was the younger girl's turn. She was very good when reminded that it was B.'s turn, though bursting with busyness. Then they changed over again, and I.S. gave a spelling test. She was very precise and particular, but very kind to us. She gathered together all the pencils and drawing-pins, etc., but lent us each a piece of rubber, "if it was for a mistake, and not carelessness." As I was rather slow, she copied mine for me, and then apparently forgot she had done so, corrected it, marked it "Ex", and gave me full marks. She did the same for B.

2. School play in which the child as teacher administers the punishments the child receives in reality.

G.W., Girl, aged 12. She became teacher; she gave me a composition lesson, then a music lesson, then drawing. Her interest shifted constantly. Worker was told to be less cheeky, neater, etc., and not to talk so much. G.W. became increasingly overbearing. She got on a chair and dropped a damp duster on worker's head. She wrote worker's name up for detention.

I.S., Girl, aged 10. (A child brought to the Institute for pilfering and backwardness.) She played a stereotyped game of a severe teacher and a stupid child. She had inexhaustible pleasure in fault-finding. Correct answers were unacceptable.

3. Altered versions of school, in which the dull child or the child who has been humiliated by failure becomes the bright one of the class.

I.S., Girl, aged 10. (She had just been put to the bottom of the class owing to apparent slackness and laziness which turned out to be due to a misunderstanding.) She was teacher and gave an excellent imitation of a good teacher, showing consideration for a slow pupil and watchfulness over a mischievous young one. She showed firmness and a sense of justice with a naughty one, but took pleasure in caning it. When another child became teacher, she was bored, and played out a game of her own, regardless of the "teacher". She became a sick child and came to school with her arm bandaged.

On another occasion. (She cannot swim.) "Daft" and "Dunce", the two rubber dolls, were giving a diving exhibition. Spectators lined the baths, before whom she showed off the prowess of her pupils. "Of course, you know, I'm the teacher", she remarked. They were made to give an exhibition of all the swimming exploits she knew of—swimming on the back, on the side, diving, and life-saving. After warning all concerned that the performance was about to finish, she made elaborate arrangements for drying "Daft" and "Dunce".

We now come to the third form of environmental play—the creation of satirical forms. When a small child throws out expressions of anger or resentment against its elders, it is apt to meet with instant retribution, and every child is very vividly aware of this fact. By the nature of the child's emotions, it is impossible for any child to prevent himself from being seized with emotions of resentment, anger, malice, and rage against the adults with whom he lives, and the knowledge that retribution will come if he expresses these emotions does not prevent his feeling them. The occurrence of such moods is neither altered nor checked by the fact that at other moments the same child feels glowing love and admiration for the same adult. Most children learn to suppress these feelings of rage by mechanisms which are too complicated to be described here. While they do succeed in repressing their main hostile emotions, the force of them cannot be entirely obliterated, and tends to break out in all sorts of unreasonable ways. When given freedom to do so, children will work the drive of these moods out of their system by giving expression to them in fantastic versions of their home and school circumstances. For example:

G.S., Girl, aged 8. She at once said I was her little girl and was to take her hand. She put her doll and its covers carefully into the pram, all the time telling me to do or not to do things, and her voice growing more and more harsh and her manner rough and nagging. She took me to the shop to buy me a toy, and told me to choose, and everything I chose she said jeeringly or crossly was unsuitable. Everything I touched she snatched out of my hand; everywhere I went, she fetched me angrily back. When I cried, she told me not to giggle; when I asked her not to be unkind, she was unmollified; but when I got into a tantrum, she relaxed at once and roared with laughter.

J.D., Boy, aged 7. He went to the dolls' house and emptied it. Then he replaced the furniture closely round the walls of three rooms, leaving the fourth empty. The two upper rooms were called "kitchen" and "bedroom", and the lower one "hospital". This contained nothing but oddments of furniture which seemed out-of-place upstairs. The fireplaces were left on the floor and some of the "world" people grouped round them, *a baby being placed inside one of the fires.* These fireplaces and the irons from the dolls' house seemed to have a special attraction for him.

R.D., Boy, aged 5. While playing with the dolls' house, he began to bathe half a dozen small pink dolls, and then he put them into a saucepan to boil. He then took three large dolls, saying one, a loose-limbed doll, was always sitting up in bed and disturbing the others. After being smacked and put back several times, she was taken across the room and buried and stamped down under a heap of overalls.

A.S., Boy, aged 7. Worker made a Girl Guide in plasticine and he smashed it up and squeezed it to nothing. (This was occasioned by the arrival of someone in uniform.) A 'queer look came over his face, the cause of which I pursued and found a "nasty" Girl Guide had teased him—as far as I could gather, for not being a Boy Scout.*

The child, in working out such plays, is in part investing the adult actors of his drama with his own emotions and in this way minimising the pressure of them within himself; partly dramatising expressions of hatred and bitterness which he really believes to be present in the adult, although more probably they exist only in himself; and partly incorporating into his play phantasy elements out of fairy-tales and myths he had heard. The examples given under Group 6 of Chapter III are also illustrative of this type of play.

All these elements act and interact in a child's environmental play. He will conduct experiments for the realisation of a part of his world, burst forth with fantastic demonstration of his conception of the nature of his world, and break into sheer burlesque of actual occurrences at home. In each he will try himself out, and, in trying himself out, come gradually to a better understanding of himself and his environment.

*During the discussion following this lecture a member of the audience quoted a normal girl of ten known to write letters to herself from an imaginary cousin, telling stories of tricking adults.

CHAPTER VII

PLAY AS PREPARATION FOR LIFE

" The plays of childhood are the germinal leaves of all later
life; for the whole man is developed and shown in these, in his
tenderest dispositions, in his innermost tendencies. The whole
later life of man, even to the moment when he shall leave it
again, has its source in the period of childhood."

FRIEDRICH FROEBEL.[38]

PROFESSOR KARL GROOS[11] has pointed out that the young of animals
play, as it were, by instinct, and that the form of their play is a rehearsal of
the rôle they are to fill in later life. Play, then, is a kind of mimic drama of
maturity, charming because of its harmlessness and purposeful in the
training it gives to the developing powers of the young animal.

As man, besides being himself, is also biologically a mammal, it would
seem to be natural that somewhere and in some way this element should
appear also in the play of children.

In his study on *The Play of Man*, Groos[12] draws particular attention to the
hunting and fighting plays of primitive peoples. Because, however, the rôles
filled by men and women in a civilised society are of such infinite variety,
and, compared to the lives and behaviour of adults in primitive societies, of
such indefinite outline from the child's point of view, one would expect it to
be difficult to trace this element clearly in the play of children of more
developed societies.

Plant life provides a useful analogy. If one could imagine an acorn to have
consciousness, there would be within it, in some dim fashion, a teleological
consciousness striving towards the minute and definite details of the tree
that is to be.

So, it would appear, must it be to some extent with the young of the
human species.

The play of children shows that the impulse to grow and develop into
specific and definite preconceived patterns exists in the vast majority of
them. The acquisition of one branch of skill seems by the very nature of the
child itself to suggest a new goal of yet greater difficulty. For instance:

" When Strumpell's little daughter learned to grasp easily," says Karl

Groos, "she was no longer satisfied with holding ordinary things, and took to picking up objects so small as to be difficult to get hold of."

This impulse to the acquisition of ever greater physical skill seems to be universal, but the form such an impulse takes is suggested to the child by the adults he sees around him, by the stories he reads, by the dreams he dreams. The play we are to consider in this chapter is the bridge between the helplessness of childhood and the possession of the power and skill for which he longs.

Throughout his work, Groos shows the existence of a definite relation between the nature of the child's struggles in play, and the type of skill and prowess he will actually need in after life.

"Play," he says, "enables the young animal to exercise himself beforehand in the strenuous and necessary functions of life, and so to be ready for their onset."

He gives examples of games whose whole purpose is the development of forms of manual skill, as for example:

"Rochholz thus describes the Swiss 'Fadmen': 'A boy sitting in a basket which is swung to and fro in the air gets a prize if he succeeds in threading a needle during the progress.'"

Every child, unless he is prohibited by his elders, tends spontaneously to evolve this sort of play for himself, and it is possible to make even the greater part of education work itself out along the lines of play.

"These familiar facts", writes Professor Percy Nunn[39], "all illuminate a single truth—namely, that the play-activity is subject to the general law that spontaneous activity, when not baffled or obstructed by unfavourable circumstances, tends always towards increasing perfection of form, to more complete expressiveness, to a higher degree of unity in diversity. Thus we are led to the idea that nature invented play not merely as a means of disposing harmlessly of the young animal's superfluous energy, but as a device for using that energy to prepare him for the serious business of life."

Such play falls into several natural divisions: motor plays, games with the senses, handcrafts, games of skill and risk, constructive plays and mental games.

Let us consider first *Motor Plays*.

We have discussed in Chapter III the child's use of his body to work off steam, to experiment with emotional states, and to demonstrate phantasy; but long ago Froebel noted the intense interest that boys take in the mere achievement of feats of bodily skill:

"The healthy boy," says Froebel[38], "brought up simply and naturally, never evades an obstacle, a difficulty; nay, he seeks it, and overcomes it.

"'Let it lie,' the vigorous youngster exclaims to his father, who is about to roll a piece of wood out of the boy's way—'let it lie; I can get over it.' With difficulty, indeed, the boy gets over it the first time; but he has accomplished the feat by his own strength. Strength and courage have grown in him. He returns, gets over the obstacle a second time, and soon learns to clear it easily. . . Hence, the daring and venturesome feats of boyhood; the explorations of caves and ravines; the climbing of trees and mountains; the searching of the heights and depths; the roaming through fields and forests. . .

"To climb a new tree means to the boy the discovery of a new world. The outlook from above shows everything so different from the ordinary cramped and distorted side-view. How clear and distinct everything lies beneath him."

Every healthy child feels a strong impulse towards experimenting with his bodily powers, and a hunger for the acquisition of curious pieces of technical skill. It is the motive upon which many systems of gymnastics are built.

Games of skill are elements in the child's progressive acquisition of control of himself or of his environment. Tennis, cricket, football, in as far as they are not work—which in modern days they so easily tend to become—are examples of this fact. As they were originally designed, a child played these games because he enjoyed them and not because he wished to win a particular trophy. It was Froebel who first laid emphasis upon the essential nature of adequate space and training in playgrounds for the development and discipline of these impulses, and who pointed out the rôle they take in the development of these qualities that he has observed to be useful in later life. He shows that this impulse to acquire the skill possessed by adults permeates child life:

"A two-year-old child of a carter", says Froebel[8], "accompanies his father and holds the horse's reins with him, firmly convinced that *he* leads the horse, and that it must obey him. A gardener's little son wishes to help his father to pull up weeds, and the father shows him how to distinguish plants by colour and scent. Another child sees his father hammering hot iron, and learns from him that the iron has been softened by the heat; or again, when he sees his father vainly attempt to push the heated bar through a hole into which it entered easily when cold, he learns that the heat has expanded the iron."

From time to time children attending the Institute experiment in the same way. For instance:

E.H., Boy, aged 4. (Father's hobby is carpentry.) He seized the bag of tools. Then he took them out one by one, asking if they were sharp. He then used the saw on pieces of wood.

On another occasion. He asked for tools, and especially the saw, and wanted to saw the handle of the hammer. He told worker to bend it, saying, " It is sharp, isn't it?" He then tried to saw with the wrong edge, insisting that this would cut too.

J.D., Boy, aged 7. (Father a porter.) He wanted to dig and was given a fork, but preferred a shovel. He is very muscular, and pulled the garden roller, lifted weights, picked up the great household box, and carried it on his head in a most professional manner.

On another occasion. He showed real concentration and energy when asked to help to tidy the room. He carried boxes, chairs, and tables about, and having asked where a chair should go, proceeded to put them all there methodically stacked.

On another occasion. Again tidying the room, he carried all the trays of sand across the room and piled them. He also carried heavy boxes of bricks, one being heaved up and carried on his head in approved porter fashion.

K.W., Boy, aged 11. (Father a carpenter and decorator.) He went to the carpenter's bench and sawed pieces of wood, holding them down with his hand and sawing extremely fast, but well and truly. He measured up the pieces frequently and very carefully.

P.T., Boy, aged 4. (Father a motor salesman.) He was attracted by the transport toys, but not interested in people or animals. He built a garage of blocks, with planks for the roof. One floor was made specially for transport vehicles.

It is a healthy sign when a child emulates that which he has observed his parents carrying out, and he will put a great deal of energy into its accomplishment.

In Chapter IV we have seen how a child will work out the recapitulation of the sensory experiences that he has already enjoyed or suffered. In older children interest in the senses looks forward rather than backwards, and takes note of the manifold uses to which the senses can be put in adult life. A child becomes interested in them, surprised or amused or occasionally repelled by them, and proceeds to experiment on his own. Let us consider what he does.

The use of the mouth offers a fascinating field for experiment to the small child. To every child it is obvious that the mouth is used by grown-ups in many ways other than for eating, and he wishes to try out what these other movements feel like, and wherein lies their charm. Whistling, making cat-calls, singing, smoking, cheering, spitting, all form part of such experimental play. Examples:

J.B., Boy, aged 6. He grabbed a little girl's toys, and then spat at worker. He climbed a ladder, and, standing on the top, tried to dislodge a spider by spitting at it. Finally he hit it, shouted with joy, and tried again.

F.V., Girl, aged 7. When worker spoke to her while she was hammering, she resented it and called worker a liar. When offered help, she spat and rebelled. She came and scribbled over worker's notebook and seemed surprised that she was not corrected. After hitting and spitting, she said, "You don't like this place, do you?"

A.U., Boy, aged 10. Four children were playing together at the Meccano table. When I came in to them, his attitude seemed to be antagonistic from the start. He spoke politely, but seemed to eye one hostilely. He was doing no work, but was leading a chorus of shrill railway whistling. He then took to whistling in the ears of two of the other children, and this led to a rough and tumble. He was given the Meccano book, but only turned it over and did not attempt to make anything. He was taken off to do something else, and after a few minutes he made one attempt to attract the others' attention by a shrill whistle across the room. But they took no notice. He gave me the impression of being out to annoy.

F.V., Girl, aged 7. She sang at the top of her voice, and screamed and yelled at worker, giving orders, countermanding them, etc. She played with a jigsaw, and sang, or rather bawled, tunes—"The Soldiers March" and "There was a Tailor had a Mouse"—but the whole time she used only the word "boo", with intermittent squawks.

Words to a small child, as we have already pointed out, do not play the same rôle as they do with the adult. They are not things of use and meaning; they stand more for sound than for meaning, and experimentation with words is one of the child's ways of growing up. Children between five and seven years of age are very much puzzled as to the meaning of words, and will take up a single word for a period of time, using it on all occasions and in reference to all kinds of objects, in order to watch the reaction of the surrounding grown-ups. They will make up nonsense rhymes and chant them as they go, and enormously enjoy the sound of shouted words.

E.C., Boy, aged 4. On entering the playroom, chanted:

> "*Here comes the boys' brigade,*
> *All covered with marmalade.*"

P.M., Boy, aged 5. While playing with the "world" toys, he referred to the hippo as the "big try horse", and, when speaking of a "world" man, he said, "He's bad, because he shoots things. He shoots men and everything—he shoots chocolate bats." He often talks nonsense language which only he can understand. When asked if anyone else can understand it, he said, "Uncle Stanley." His nonsense words nearly always rhyme. The following are examples: "Big spanky bead bocky." "Big bumping father." "Mr. Big rude booby."

Another use of the mouth which fascinates children is its capacity to produce tastes. This interest is not universal, but it persistently appears in a certain number of children. They have noticed the variety of tastes the world can supply, and find the quality and taste of substances of endless interest, inventing numberless ingenious games to try them out. The following are examples:

B.G., Boy, aged 9. While blowing bubbles, he said it tasted like pineapple and was nice.

On another occasion. He told worker that he liked pudding, especially bread pudding. He always has a "whacking great helping". He also liked meat, because "when you cough after eating it, you taste it again."

On another occasion. He was biting his nails while reading. Worker enquired what it felt like, and he replied, "Oh, it tastes ever so good."

P.T., Boy, aged 4. While playing with the mincer, he first began mincing, then he took it to pieces and screwed it up. He cut plasticine into strips to feed it. His interest then passed to cutting the plasticine into ever thinner strips, and at times he handed bits to worker to bite, asking, "Does it taste nasty?" He was thrilled by this, but did not dare to bite it himself.

Stanley Hall[13] quotes some interesting examples of children experimenting with the use of the mouth:

"F., 4. Wanted to taste horseradish, and, being refused, tasted it when her mother's back was turned.

"F., 4. Was very curious about a box of paris green and narrowly escaped poisoning.

"F., 4, and M., 4½. Tasted grafting wax but did not like the flavour.

"F., 4. Ate raw potato to see how it tasted.

"M., 6, and F., 8. My sister and I used to mix up snow and milk and juices to make new drinks.

"F., 6. Ate green grapes to see if they would really make her sick, as she had been told.

" M., 6. Tasted Tabasco sauce, although he had been warned of the effect."

A variety of this interest in taste is the boys' and girls' interest in substitutes for cigarettes. Stanley Hall writes:

" Mr. Bell gives a list of seventy-one different substances tested as to their smoking qualities by boys and girls of these ages. Bark of various kinds, spices, seeds, leaves, stems, rattan, cork—in fact, almost anything that could be smoked and was easily procurable—is to be found in this list. While it is undoubtedly true that imitation plays a large part in this smoking craze, its root lies in the natural desire of growing children to test new sensations for themselves, and even the unpleasant results consequent upon some of the trials do not prevent further experimentation along the same line."

Visual experiments are more rare, but every child at one time or another bandages its eyes and plays games with itself or with its friends, to investigate the meaning of sight—no sight, pressing eyeballs to see "stars", squinting, shutting alternate eyes. Experiments with colour selection comes under this head. The following are examples of children showing interest in visual effects:

B.H., Girl, aged 8. She saw another girl painting wood in a dirty yellow colour. She said she disliked the colour intensely, but wanted to paint wood. The only other colour available at the time was blue. She tired of using this, and decided that she liked the yellow better after all. On another day she used orange, put it on very thickly, and remarked that " it looks like chalk when it is dry."

D.D., Girl, aged 10. When making a picure with Čizek material she chose rather sombre colours with a certain tastefulness.

D.J., Girl, aged 11. Using "concentration" toy, she made a flowing design, then took it to pieces and arranged the material in long rows of uniform colours side by side. She expressed decided preference for blue and less marked liking for green.

B.C., Girl, aged 10. When cutting out and sticking pictures into a book, she showed marked preference for blue, which is associated with blue dress, shoes, stockings, coat, hat. " My sister made the blue dress I've got. Blue for beauty." Worker asked, " What do you see that is blue?" and she replied, " The sky is blue, but I never look at it."

Experiments with smell also occur, but are difficult to illustrate. These examples show a dislike of certain smells:

M.R., Girl, aged 11. Another girl had found a scent-bottle and insisted upon sprinkling the scent on her clothes and toys. She said that she disliked scent and grimaced in disgust.

B.C., Girl, aged 10. She expressed sharp dislike of the smell of gum. Worker tried to suggest things it was like, but failed. The following afternoon the discussion of the smell of glue was resumed.*

Next we come to experimentation with external objects. On page 149, we have referred to an example given by Froebel of the child's delight in overcoming obstacles, and even creating them in order to overcome them.

Children when left to themselves will spontaneously set themselves constructive tasks of ever-increasing difficulty, and will show an almost incredible power of absorption in these tasks, and patience in the steady overcoming of difficulties which often exceeds anything ever again realised in later life.

Charlotte Bühler[20] has brought out a very important point in regard to this relationship between the child and its material:

"The child progresses in this development from the primitive forms of pleasure in activity", she writes, "to pleasure in creation, a specifically human pleasure experience which first appears with the construction of an object. In contrast to the pleasure of activity, in which we pour forth our energy in movements, we have in the pleasure of creation the characteristic satisfaction of transferring our energy to the material, and of impressing upon it the stamp of our individuality. We generally express this by saying that we express ourselves in the material. And in this expression of ourselves we expand beyond our limits and leave a more or less permanent impression of ourselves in the material. With this are connected three important experiences characteristic of mankind . . . while he is active with the material, man surrenders himself to it, masters it, and puts something new into the world. Surrendering one's self, mastering the material, and producing an object are, one may say, such definitely human experiences that without them one is not human. These experiences . . . have normally fallen to the lot of the six-year-old child."

Without such a surrendering, and the capacity to make such a surrender, normal emotional and character growth cannot take place. Children, deprived of adequate opportunities of constructive play, are children who later grow up deficient in constructive imagination, and are inhibited in experience.

Charlotte Bühler is of the opinion that the passage from the use of

*During the discussion following this lecture a member of the audience quoted girls of eleven to twelve known to show great interest in smelling different herbs in a garden and comparing their scents.

material as an instrument for phantasy to the use of even the same material for construction, is a definite stage in maturation. While the age-limits she suggests and the fixity of the lines she draws cannot be entirely accepted as universally applicable, it is without doubt that a desire to construct makes its appearance in all healthy children at a definite period. Constructive play is a constant feature of work in the Institute playroom, and the constructive material has heavy demands made upon it by children of all ages. Here are a few records:

E.H., Boy, aged 3¾. He wanted to make "a push-chair for my baby". He examined the basket of tools, and took out the saw and used it. He then looked for the pincers and for a "thing like my dad has" (plane). He picked up a large hammer and held it for a few moments, then threw it down and returned to his small one. He continued his work more and more independently; at first it was, "You do it; you hold it", but later he pushed worker's hand away, saying, "I'll do it."

On another occasion. He said, "Let's make a ladder what a man can go up. You do it." Worker showed him how to put the pieces together, and began the ladder. He snatched it away and with a chuckle pushed the rungs apart. Then he pulled it to pieces and put it away. He asked what was in the various boxes, and finally accepted the component parts of an airship. He began working on this, and was absorbed, but asked continually, "Is it finished?" Before completion, it was rejected in favour of an aeroplane and a ship of painted wood. He was interested in fitting pieces together, but did not attempt to make anything, nor did the pictures of the completed models interest him. He specially liked the funnel. He then passed on to very simple "motor" construction. This he completed with a good deal of help, and showed great satisfaction. He wanted to show it to his mother. In working at this, he was very quick in picking up and adopting information given in answer to his questions.

A.J., Boy, aged 7. He asked for the match-box construction game, and began to make a train, working very steadily at it, but choosing on the whole the easier parts of the construction. It was amusing to note that although he insisted upon worker doing all the difficult parts, he continually stated to her in question form, "I did do it all, didn't I?"

J.W., Boy, aged 14. He wanted to build something, and, after surveying all the printed construction plans, slowly chose a crane. He seemed loth to have a plan dictated to him, but at the same time unaccustomed to the idea of choosing one himself. Save for one detail, his design followed the printed plan. At one point he asked worker, "Is that right?"

On another occasion. On arrival he asked, "Can I finish the thing I started last time?" We found the crane and he settled down. He was very silent, and worked hard and intelligently. He asked once if the model was going all right, and from time to time tested the crane, and was worried to find it rickety. When it was finished, he wanted something heavy to tie on to it for it to lift.

I.K., Boy, aged 13. He looked through the constructive play materials, and found the model of a motor-car which consisted of only a few pieces, and was fairly easy. He said, " I don't want this sort of thing. This is already done for you; there is nothing left for you to do." He then became interested in a fire-engine model and decided to do it. Before even beginning work, he discovered that pieces were lacking. Worker found substitutes and he then started to work. He looked at the picture of the model and said that he did not want to copy it. He liked to make something of his own, or to improve on the model. Later he remarked, " Actually I mean to say I am almost certain to improve on the model." He fastened two wheels on an iron rod, and then discovered that the model engine was out of proportion and made an elaborate proof of this statement, and went on to talk of proportions generally.

Handcraft. The function which construction fulfils for boys is fulfilled for girls in the main by handcraft. But this division is not in any way absolute. The fascination of punching needles through cards, and the permanence of the pattern that can be left; the fun of altering the appearance of a doll by changing its dress; and the delight of beadwork, are fascinations that are felt equally by boys and girls at any early age, and many more boys than the few who do would retain, and would exercise, if custom permitted it, this same interest in later life. Here are examples of girls' interest in handcraft:

D.S., Girl, aged 12. I helped her remove from the loom the bead square she had finished weaving and prepare the purse it was to decorate. When she had finished this purse, she appeared decidedly happier than before, showing more easiness and spontaneity in her attitude to work, children, and workers, and making better contact with them. She was obviously pleased with having done her weaving well, and started gleefully swinging by supporting herself between the chair and the table.

I.S., Girl, aged 9. She was cutting out pictures and pasting, and worker asked if she would like to make a Christmas card for her mother. She was very pleased with the idea, but thought a calendar would be nicer. She was very enthusiastic over her work, and demanded that others should see it and appreciate it.

M.E., Girl, aged 14. She was sewing a plain yellow line, and several times undid several parts of it, stitching backwards, as there were mistakes. Having finished her yellow row, she began another row in blue, carefully showing me the colour. I had to prepare new threads, etc., for her, and she refused to take a thread again, once it had been pulled out. She asked for permission to take her handwork home, as she wanted to "finish all this".

On another occasion. I showed her the embroidery I had started with another girl, and she decided to finish this, each of us to do one end, and it was to be a competition of speed. The attitude of "mother and child" game was deliberately chosen, and she forbade me to speak until I had finished my work. When both our pieces of work were finished, she asked if she might take them home.

Handcraft has for girls naturally a technical side, and a side that is not play, but lies in the region of work. Where the little boy is interested in the tools of the trade exercised by his father, the little girl makes beds, mixes dough, sews dolls' clothes, not this time to release her energy or to "take her mother off", but in order to acquire the kind of skill that mummy has.

In small children play with the materials of domestic life is recapitulatory play, phantasy play, or sense experiment; in adults, it is work or artistic creation. In the girl of junior and middle school age there should come, if her development in this side of her nature is going to follow the lines of natural growth, a period of contact with the raw materials of her future domestic occupations, in the form of play and not work. This play is preparation for life, in the sense that the achievements the child has seen brought about in adult life are actually attempted and studied, but the relative emphasis which is put upon achievement of experiment should be left entirely to her own initiative. That is to say, she should be allowed to cook with the cook, or in cookery classes, making *play* cookery of her own and copying the actions of the cook as best as she can, but being allowed to break off now and then to elaborate the games suggested by the chance shape of the piece of rolled pastry, or the position of two currants as the eyes of a monster. In the end she will produce perhaps one cake which is near enough to the real thing to be accepted by the cook, to the great delight of the child, and put among her own productions. It may be objected that to allow a child to do this is merely to allow her to waste materials, but the answer is that if children are given the chance to become familiar for themselves, in their own way, with the natural qualities of the materials used, for example, in cookery, they will bring ultimately to the learning of actual cookery the same zest and interest that they bring to their play.

Play with iron, steel, and oil in the garage, in the ship-builders' yard, in the fisheries, in the carpenter's shop, in the piggeries and the stables of the farm perform for the boy the same function as this type of domestic play performs for the girl. Such play eases the junction between childhood and maturity; softens the passage from fantastic living to living in contact with reality; and, if successful in fortunate circumstances, children brought up in this way carry over into the mature, skilful constructive ability of the grown man and woman something of the imaginative and creative power of the child. Here are examples of the kind of play that is meant:

G.S., Girl, aged 8. She went to play with dough, and put flour into three basins and then added water to each. At first she made firm pies, then sloshier ones, and one that became accidentally pink she made more so with chalk and called it tomato soup. She added handfuls of fine sand, calling it salt. She then made another large basin of sand and water, and thought worker stupid because she did not recognise it as coffee.

L.F., Girl, aged 8. Playing with house material, she put "potatoes" on to boil. Then she put a kettle of water on to boil and went to the lavatory, telling worker to take the kettle off when it boiled. On her return she accused worker of taking some of the water and not leaving her enough for a cup of tea.

A.J., Boy, aged 5. (Father a blacksmith.) He spent some time hammering nails into wood, and showed a remarkable skill with the hammer, hitting nails well on the head in a masterly fashion. If one was driven in crooked, he hit it on the side to straighten it.

Games of Risk. Here appears a very important element in life. Risk and danger are a normal element of adult life, and the ability to cope with dangerous situations is a mark of successful adult character. Every child has a hunger to emulate in this way the adults who surround him, and every child, if left to itself, will create games in which the element of risk apears.

In his section on "Direct Physical Fighting Play", Groos[12] described children provoking or inviting one another to fight:

"So far as my observation goes in this little investigated sphere, very small boys seldom stand for their combats. Usually one already seated seizes his comrade, who may be standing near, by the foot, pulls him down, and they fight, rolling over on the floor, and each seeking to keep the upper hand. The effort is constantly made to keep the enemy's head down, a position so distasteful to the party concerned that the scene threatens to end in noisy and serious strife. . . Usually the fight ends at this point, but sometimes the tussling is continued on the ground, as described, and the playful character is very apt to be lost. . . The enjoyment is doubled when it becomes not only a question of hitting the enemy, but of dodging his missiles as well."

Groos clearly shows that he recognises the desire to take risks or to provoke them, if they are absent, although he does not appear to have attached a great importance to the desire to take risks *per se*. This universal desire is shown in the play at the I.C.P.:

J.B., Boy, aged 7. While in the garden he climbed the fig-tree and picked the small green figs. Then he found a pile of twigs near a tree. He climbed up these and stood on the wall, looking on to the roof of the staff cloakroom. He asked if he might climb on the roof, but worker said it would be very disturbing to people inside, so he agreed to come down. He climbed the fig-tree again, and was delighted to see people watching from the parents' room. He hoped " mum " was there; " she wouldn't half be frightened."

E.R., Boy, aged 11. He climbed up the flag-staff at the end of the garden, and found a rope down which he climbed. Then, seeing a metal wire, he said, " I'm going to walk the rope."

He lassoed worker, and plants, sticks, etc.

This element in children's nature forms one of the most serious obstacles to the achievement of safety for children in modern streets and roads. There is a game of " Last Across ", which has always had a fascination for children. This could be played with reasonable safety while the traffic consisted of horses and carts—it is rare for a horse to tread on a human being—but lorries have no such sensibility. Moreover, a small child has a besetting difficulty in distinguishing animate from inanimate objects, and particularly in relation to movement, and finds it impossible to appreciate the deadliness of moving lorries.

Contributory to this delight is that of boarding moving objects. The boarding of a moving vehicle holds an irresistible attraction for every unsophisticated boy. To mount up beside the milkman, to ride in the lorry, or to be taken up beside the driver of a heavy commercial vehicle, is an achievement beside which all risks pale into insignificance. From the days of Buffalo Bill to the present day there remains this powerful impulse in healthy childhood, and it is an impulse which, if it does not succeed in gaining reasonable scope, or if it is unduly inhibited by fear, tends to weaken the spirit of enterprise throughout the child's character. On this impulse the Boy Scout movement, the Sea Scouts, the success of boys' and girls' camps, and of Alpine parties for boys and girls are largely based.

The thrill which underlies games in which risk is involved is very closely associated with the emotions of suspense and fear. Many children intensely enjoy games involving a certain moderate element of fear. As, for example:

" A little girl of seven related in a very animated manner that she and her sister loved to feel frightened. ' We love to play with the fire; it may burn us—but we don't care; we love to be frightened. We love to swing high in the swing—it frightens us—we love it.' " (Privately contributed.)

Also the recollection of a friend whose childhood was spent in Spain:

" We used to love to bathe in a pool that was set out of bounds by our parents' command. We would dip our feet in the pool, and swing down on the branches and get wet, fearful and delighted by the excitement and fear that our disobedience produced, not, I may say, by the chance of any activity on the part of the alligators that infested the pool."

Instances of this kind have been noted by many observers of children. It is as if the child were testing the lengths to which its endurance of the pleasurable qualities inherent in fear would go, and testing out its own capacities for sensation. This joy continues throughout adult life, and reappears in adult delight in gangster films and thriller plays and books. The creation of situations containing strong emotion in a safe atmosphere, where the player knows beforehand that no real disaster can happen, is one of the most permanent elements of the play sense of mankind.

Closely akin to the joy in taking physical risk is the delight most healthy children feel in the exercise of mental agility. Roughly around the age of ten years, energy begins to pour into mental processes, and the healthy child, finding school work an insufficient outlet for its energy, invents mental tests and trials of skill of his own.

Into this group come guessing games, riddles, arithmetic games, games of observation, and games played with paper and pencil.

Groos[12], unfortunately, in his section on mental plays gives very few examples of children's experiments with their mental faculties, but does, in the following extract, describe a self-devised guessing game of a very small child:

"Marie G., who from the time she was two years old had a veritable passion for having things drawn for her, considered it a great joke when she could not make out what was meant without some effort."

In the I.C.P. from time to time during their stay, and at the end of their period of attendance, when the children are gaining some freedom from the tyranny of their own emotional problems, they invent games of experiment with their mental powers. For example:

A.M., Boy, aged 13. He made out and exhibited with pride a code which he said he used in his classroom with a friend who sits behind him.

B.G., Boy, aged 11. He wanted to write something for the sake of writing, but did not know what to do. He decided to write out the capitals of Europe, saying that in school you could not take so much care and time.

M.B., Girl, aged 12. She suggested making words from a long word, and agreed to use the word "incompatibility".

G.W., Girl, aged 12. She suggested a title for the story we were both to write, i.e., "A Terrible Disaster."

G.W.: "I will give you marks and you shall give me marks. Of course, yours will be best."

Worker: " But I can't spell, and spelling faults take off marks."

G.W.: " I can spell and I shall count every fault against you."

On another occasion. She asked to do spelling, and worker had to select long words as a test of her spelling ability.

On yet another occasion. She was looking for "difficult words " and was very scornful at worker's failure to find words she did not know. She stumbled occasionally, but only in the case of words that were not likely to be familiar to her.*

This interest passes on later into crossword puzzles and the interest which is so widespread in complicated detective fiction.

It is an interesting fact to note how the children of artists experiment in painting, the children of mathematicians either hate or take premature interest in mathematical problems, and how the children of writers fill countless copybooks with stories and plays of their own. " All work without play makes Jack a dull boy ", and the modern educationalist has come to see that the elimination of play from education greatly lessens a child's capacity to learn, and that play itself is a valuable and indispensable vehicle of learning.[40]

" No candid observer ", says Sir Percy Nunn[39], " can doubt that school teaching would be immensely more efficient if teachers could learn to exploit the intellectual energy released so abundantly in play."

*During the discussion following this lecture a member of the audience quoted the desire to do long sums at seven years and to add them up, and the joy in juggling with figures.

CHAPTER VIII

GROUP GAMES

"In every case the plays of this age are, or should be, pure manifestations of strength and vitality; they are the product of fullness of life, and of pleasure in life. They presuppose actual vigour of life, both inner and outer. Where these are lacking, there cannot be true play, which, bearing life in itself, awakens, nourishes, and heightens life."

FROEBEL.
Froebel and Modern Psychology.

MANY COLLECTIONS have been made of the group games of children, and in the view of many observers these constitute the main form of play in childhood. Such collections are rarely analysed into types, but among the games noted the following classes can be distinguished:

GAMES OF A TRADITIONAL FORM ASSOCIATED WITH MELODY AND RHYME

Many theories are rife regarding the origin of the traditional singing games of childhood. The general opinion is that they are the minute fragments that remain of ceremonies that were at one time general among adults. Certainly this is true of the "Herody" played by Polish children at Christmas-time, and of other folk-plays of this kind which partake more of the nature of drama, and are clearly themselves debased morality plays.

Games of this type are spread all over the world, and perhaps the best studies of national groups are Roth's study of the games of North Queensland children[41], and Culin's of the children of Korea[42]. Some games show a very wide distribution, for example, "Ring-a-ring of Roses". Others are strictly local, but all are handed down either from adults or from older children to the younger, and the strict tradition is maintained by each generation. On the whole, traditional singing games are played more by younger than by the rather older children.

GAMES INVOLVING RUNNING, CHASING, AND CAPTURE

There is an infinite variety of games of this sort; they range from such as "Fill up the Gap" and "Twos and Threes", played mostly by middle school hildren, to such as "Hunt the Slipper", which may be played at any age. The characteristic of these games is the splitting of the group into three elements, the chaser, the chased (even if the chased is represented by a slipper), and the excited, watching crowd.

Games involving Make-believe Combat and a Division into Sides

These may be arranged so that the game is all against one as in those of he type of "Steps" and "Blind Man's Buff", "Mushrooms", and "Tom Tiddler's Ground"; or half the group may be arrayed against the other half, as in "French and English", "Prisoners and Flags".

Here the game has more form. Sides have to be "picked up" in some of hem; some give scope for leadership; and in others for a moment all the imelight is concentrated upon a single child who pits his skill against the rest.

Guessing Games

"Up, Jenkins", "Forfeits", "Charades", "Dumb Crambo", and a hundred other types of game in which the essential is the pitting of the wits of one part of the group against the skill of the other. These games can be active, as in "Charades"; partly active, as in "Up Jenkins"; or entirely silent, as in "Dumb Crambo".

Games of Intellectual Skill and Agility

Here come in all the board and pieces games—"Draughts", "Halma", "Chess", "Pegity", "Fox and Geese", with "Dominoes" as a distant cousin, and the card games, "Happy Families", "Rummy", and "Snap", in all its varieties, and many of the games with ordinary cards. In this group should also be included the infinite variety of games which are played with paper and pencil.

Games of Chance

Here we have the numberless games that are played with dice, with balls and numbers, and with playing-cards. Opportunity to play games of this kind seems to be craved by every little boy or girl at one age or another, and most children pass through a stage of concentrated absorption in them, which seems to give them a satisfaction to be gained in no other way.

An interesting study has been made by Hildegard Hetzer[43] of children playing games in the streets of Kaisermühlen, and the games of London children have been collected in *Street Games*.

From the days of Froebel, it has been agreed that taking part in group games is a necessary part of a child's life. Froebel held that rhyme and song

are an essential part of these games, and that the moving together o
children in an ordered way, fulfilling a ritual set down in the dim ages of the
past and carrying no personal flavour, brings to a child a sense of corporate
being, a sense of a life larger than his own. If he can give himself to materia
in construction, he can give himself to a game, and in identification with the
material or the group's game find a temporary rest from his own problems
an outlet for his energies, and a satisfaction for his social sense.

But there are other forms of games which are also played in groups and
do not come under this classification, namely:

FORMLESS ROUGH AND TUMBLE

" Let's have a rough house ", says a fifteen-year-old boy, enjoying the force
of muscle against muscle for its own sake. Tumbling over one another
shapeless wrestling matches, and horse-play forms a group by itself in the
play of older children, analogous to the " letting off steam " of the five- to
six-year-olds. Here are illustrations culled from the Institute records:

A.M., Boy, aged 13, and M.E., Girl, aged 14. M.E. climbed on the boy's back
and slid over his head on to the floor. This was repeated two or three
times, each being rather rough with the other.

A.M., Boy, aged 13, B.G., Boy, aged 11, and G.W., Girl, aged 13. They acted a
play made up by themselves. Each one came in in turn, picked up a
newspaper, read it, and collapsed in a faint on the floor. A.M. fell on top
of G.W., and a scrimmage followed, each trying to push the others out.
saying " This is *my* house." Much enjoyment shown by all.

This kind of play is of the same nature as " ragging "; and delight in
" ragging " persists well into the early twenties.

Opportunity for rough and varied play of this kind is almost a necessity
for a healthy adolescence. So many odd and shifting moods can be
expressed in this way, and by expression brought within the lad's or girl's
power of control, that they subserve a very valuable purpose in development, and nothing else quite takes their place.

UNORGANISED GROUP GAMES

These are intermediate between rough-and-tumble movements of the
" rough house " type and the organised games we have considered. They are
the shadow of organised games such as football and cricket, but are played
with shifting rules. The general scheme follows the lines of the real game,
but the rules continually alter as it appears to the players that the exigencies
of the game demand. Such games serve as an escape from the rigidity of
rules, and make a bridge between loose phantasy games and the organised
" games " of the public school. Were it natural to children to play to

ermanent and unchanging rules, the importance of cricket and football oaches in our schools would not be as obvious as it is, and "games" would e a far more spontaneous part of school life. In the nursery the very young hild displays an "alarming" disregard for rules, and likes to play its active nd sitting games in its own way, a way which results in a running earrangement of rules to make the game easier or more interesting for the layer. Later on such alteration is called "cheating", and becomes one of the einous crimes of childhood. The Institute records provide many examples f such games. Here is a typical one:

G.W., *Girl, aged 13½.* She was playing with a boy and two workers, and agreed to "Rounders". The two children picked partners. It was a most peculiar game, and G.W. appointed herself mistress of ceremonies. What she said was law, and, although we all disagreed with her rulings, she would not listen to us and insisted upon having her own way. The game got completely out of hand, both children becoming more and more aggressive.

REPRESENTATIONAL GAMES

These have been considered in Chapter III from the activity side, and in Chapter V from the side of the phantasy expressed. It remains here to consider them as expressions of corporate playing or group games. The essence of games of this kind is the formation of spontaneous groups to carry out a group idea. The characters usually chosen are pirates, gangsters, kings and queens, and adventurers, and the material from which these plots are drawn comes from boys' and girls' school magazines, fairy-tales, nursery rhymes, films, history, and traditional forms. Usually the form of the game is reinforced by the fascination of dressing up. Examples:

C.B., *Boy, aged 10,* G.T., *Boy aged 7, and* I.C., *Girl, aged 9.* I.C. and G.T. wanted a procession, C.B. to make the music. Suddenly they discovered the acting clothes, and they all wanted to dress up, getting very excited about it. C.B. took the sword-belt and looked for something to use as a sword. He made drum music for the King and Queen to come in, and then put a crown on his head and said that he was the right King and G.T. was a traitor. He wanted to fight him with his sword, but worker prevented this and suggested a decision by trial, another worker to be the judge. The Queen was asked, and said that C.B. was the right King. G.T. agreed, saying he was a foreign King on a visit. A feast was given for him, and C.B. and I.C. danced, not listening to the gramophone music, but making a great deal of noise with their tambourines.

After G.T. had gone, C.B. and I.C. decided that they were King and Queen of Italy, for which purpose they changed and dressed up again carefully behind the screen. Sometimes C.B. was King and sometimes Chancellor,

and he was a peaceful King. Then they went to bed, and worker was told
to be the servant and to bring them a scarf or coat for them to wear a
night clothes, or to use as blankets. She was to call them in the morning
and provide breakfast, which the King ordered as if in a hotel, and to
fetch the newspaper, etc. There was a string of pearls on the floor, which
worker was ordered to find, and not to deliver. The Queen then found
the pearls in worker's pocket, called her a traitor, and dismissed her, but
on worker's appeal for pardon, it was granted by the King.
C.B. asked who was the man who took off his coat so that the Queen might
walk on it, and said that he was that man. They then acted the scene.
G.T. came back again as a visiting King. The King and Queen danced.
Suddenly C.B. said that the red rug was his coffin because he was going to
war and would die. He bade farewell to the Queen and went off to the war
(lavatory). He came back wounded, knocking at the door, and was laid on
the rug and the doctor (G.T.) was fetched. C.B., being wounded in the
chest, wanted to have the bullet taken out and the wound dressed. (He
said he was bleeding all over.) G.T. ordered him only to stay in bed and
have nothing to eat but orange juice, but finally a dressing was made. The
Queen was not allowed to see him, or to come into the room next door or
opposite, as she might "catch it". C.B. was very quiet and patient
speaking in a faint voice. Then he recovered, got up, went out, and
suddenly fell dead. He was then put in the coffin and buried. I.C. then
married G.T., but C.B. suddenly came to life again (at I.C.'s suggestion)
and called G.T. a traitor.

C.B. and R.S., both Boys, aged 10. Worker was told to be a Princess and to get
all the pearls, jewels, beads, and nice things she could find. The Princess
was moved by coach from Buckingham Palace to Windsor Castle; and on
the way attacked by C.B. and R.S., and taken away in an "extra cell" of
their coach to Africa, where she would be eaten by lions. The Princess
offered a ransom which her husband would pay, and they then went away
and killed the husband.

*H.F. and A.M., Boys, aged 13, R.S., Boy, aged 10, O.M., Girl aged 12, and I.C.,
Girl, aged. 9.* H.F. at the piano was making music representing the sea.
A.M. was Captain, R.S. a sailor (complete with sword-belt), O.M. the
captain's wife, first worker a grumbling old lady, and second worker a
stewardess.
H.F. played a storm, sometimes teasing A.M. by saying he played the captain
speaking. Then they were all seasick. R.S. shouted, "Man overboard",
and the captain went to rescue him. They were then all dead, but H.F.
wanted them to come to life again, and A.M. played wildly at the piano.
Later I.C. was Queen, A.M. King, R.S. a soldier, H.F. a "boozer", O.M. a
servant, two workers were daughters (at O.M.'s request).
The drunkard attacked the soldier; then the soldier and the King fought

together against him. They made him prisoner, A.M. being very aggressive against H.F. and wanted to tie him up. Then they locked him in the water-room.

The second act was supposed to represent the court. Meanwhile H.F., who seemed rather upset, hammered against the door , and when the others opened it they said the prisoners had gone mad and that nobody could go in there. The two servants went to fetch him, and found him with a stick, hammer, and saw which he wanted to take with him. The servants said that no arms were allowed in court. In court the prisoner said he was going to fire the palace and kill the King, and that all the people in the country were supporting him. He attacked the guard, and then there was another fight, R.S. and A.M. against H.F.

M.E., Girl, aged 14, and F.V., Girl, aged 7. The preparations and dressing up took a very long time behind the curtains. F.V. wore trousers and wings, and M.E. a fantastic female gown and a mask with a lace veil.

The two children appeared several times, on each occasion saying the same words, "It seems to me that this is an enchanted wood." After a long pause they again appeared and explained that there was a nightingale sitting on a tree—it had been sitting there for many hours. They walked beneath the tree and found a letter which the nightingale had dropped. M.E. with great difficulty (very well acted) read it to F.V. The letter stated that they were to go by aeroplane or by ship to visit a Princess.

On the way to visit the Princess, they found they were very thirsty. Although previously warned by the nightingale to avoid beer, they disregarded his advice, and M.E. fell drunk and fainted. F.V. brought her water, which she managed to drink, in spite of the difficulties of negotiating with her veil.

They have apparently separated, and meet in a wood, F.V. carrying a rubber tube as a revolver.

F.V.: "Your money or your life!"

M.E.: "Have you some change?"

F.V. has not, so they fight, M.E. being the victor. F.V., lying on the floor, begged her pardon and promised to say who she is. M.E. allowed her to get up, and she then refused to give the information. As a punishment, M.E. tore off her wings, explaining that she was no longer a Prince (or a Princess).

Same two children on another occasion. M.E. grabbed F. V., and rushed through the playroom, saying, "Come on, we're going to act a play." They spent a considerable time behind the curtain, and at last appeared to act "Jack and Jill". M.E. was Jack, wearing a red dressing-gown and a paper headdress. Jack asked Jill to help him get the water, so they climbed the hill and then fetched a bucket, but it was full of sand, so they took it back and fetched a large basin of water, Jack blaming Jill all the time. They spilt some water, and then both rolled on the floor.*

A great deal of study has been given to the social impulses of children, and there is considerable difference of opinion as to the age at which social play becomes possible.

Piaget[32] sees the child as beginning in an autistic phase, and puts the appearance of language as a consequence of the development of the social phase. Susan Isaacs[31] criticises this, and regards the social life of children as a gradual development from the earliest years. Hidegard Hetzer[43] states that from two to three years 100 per cent of the children in the streets of Kaisermühlen played only with grown-ups; in the fourth year they began to be absorbed into group games of two, three, and four older children; and in the sixth year there predominated games of three and four children. She noticed also that for the smaller children watching and imitation of older children formed the major part of their social contacts, but from ten years on they began mostly to originate games of their own, details of which are given in the following table.

Age in Years	Sex Boy Girl	No Set Play	Co-operation and Imitation	Set Play	Free Play	Percent-age
3	♂ and ♀	33	50	17	—	100
4–6	♂ and ♀	16	30	51	3	100
6–10	♂ and ♀	2	18	60	20	100
10–15	♂	—	10	23	67	100
10–15	♀	—	16	25	59	100

A former student of the I.C.P. notes in regard to normal four-year-olds of which she is in charge:

" Betty and Elizabeth are playing ' Families '. Elizabeth is ' Baby ', and is sat in a box and covered with a cloth by Betty. Betty goes away to the ' kitchen ', then comes back and puts Elizabeth on a trolley and pushes her off. They talk about their play and Betty tells Elizabeth what to do.

" Peter, Tony, and Billie have two trains and a large station house, with a bridge entrance. They push their trains in and build up the walls with

---

*During the discussion following this lecture a member of the audience quoted a child of three and a half known to act Cinderella by herself to herself. Another child of two acted fairy-tales made up by herself, taking all the parts herself.

Another member quoted children of five in her kindergarten acting a story made up by themselves about frog families.

Another member quoted children of three and a half playing " Pop goes the Weasel " on their own initiative—directed by a child of four.

bricks. Bertie pushes his train up and into the house and then goes off on to his own play. The others continue at intervals, and the walls grow higher and higher until they finally topple over."

In I.C.P. records, impulses towards sociability are found as early as the age of two and a half years—for instance, in the following example—but they are fleeting and spasmodic.

T.B., Boy, aged 2½. He played quite nicely with a boy aged 3 years; although he tends to want to take things from the others, the impulse is spasmodic. He wanted to take away the things the others had, saying "Tommy's, Tommy's", but generally became attached to worker. He seemed jealous of the other children, and several times fetched me away from them to play with him.

Professor Bridges' elaborate study of the social life of the pre-school child[28] corroborates the variability of the reactions of the very young child. The following are examples from Institute records:

N.T., Girl, aged 2. She was very interested in the other children, particularly in one boy, and she laughed at the noises he made. She was very suspicious, and, I think, inclined to be jealous of another little boy—she watched him out of the corner of her eye.

On another occasion. M.M. and his sister came in when she had just started playing, and she obviously resented their taking up worker's attention. She was also very much annoyed when the little boy poured water on to her tray, or tried to take her things. After playing with the dolls' pram, she left it and said, "Hello", to another girl through the "shop" window. She took the ducks from M.M.'s sand tray and gave them to worker, then put them on the floor. These seemed to give her great joy. She took a handful of the red sticks that M.M. had been playing with, and went upstairs to the parents' room with them and refused to come down again, saying, "No, no."

K.W., Boy, aged 2½. He and another boy played with toy animals, but he was rather inclined to want anything the other had. He then started deliberately teasing him by throwing his mosaic squares into the box. H. took this very well and quite patiently turned them out—then K.W. took to hitting him, and shouting for joy, but when worker said, "Oh, poor Harry!" he stopped at once.

On another occasion. On his own initiative he put all the things back in the cupboard, and chose a doll which he carried round for some time, but left when fresh bricks were given to him. He pointed out the pictures on the cupboard and told me the bird was a parrot. He played with another child and made a long train with bricks—his own suggestion—which he pushed along. He played most contentedly all the time, whether alone or with two older children who played with him.

Here are examples of sociability in children up to six years:

E.H., Boy, aged 4. He made advances to other boys of his own size, holding out things to them from his own supply and giving them to worker, saying, "You give that to that little boy."

On another occasion. To-day he was conversational and reasonable. He accepted me as a playfellow, giving me my share of each toy and equal opportunities. He wished to make things and show that he could.

P.T., Boy, aged 4. He and another little boy played together with a large aluminium airship and large bricks. They built a garage and ran the airship up and down the room, and into it. They perfectly understood and agreed about taking turns at this, and spoke to each other.*

After this age the picture is profoundly affected by a variety of factors which are to be considered in Chapter X.

Apart from the question of age, as has already been said, the neurotic child rarely combines with his fellows—he will sit apart in the middle even of a group of children absorbed in group play, and continue with his own activity, playing with himself inside his mind, if he is playing at all, and totally unable to combine with those outside.

To be able to play in a group, certain particular qualities of personality are necessary, and it is the exercise of these characteristics that creates the enjoyment of group games. Such qualities are:

A SPONTANEOUS DESIRE FOR ASSOCIATION WITH OTHER HUMAN BEINGS

No group game can arise unless the children composing it are at that moment more interested in the feeling of association with other children than in the experiments or plays they are carrying out by themselves. That is to say, to use the terms created by Dr. Jung, they must be at that moment more extraverted than introverted. The emphasis in a group game is

---

*During the discussion following this lecture a member of the audience quoted two three-year-olds in her nursery school playing mother and baby, talking together quite reasonably.

Another member of the audience quoted from her infant school small children talking together, discussing toys, etc., while waiting for the marking of the register.

Another member of the audience quoted a firm friendship known to exist between three-year-olds.

Another member of the audience quoted a boy of two and a half to three years entirely dominating another child, a boy of mixed race.

basically more on association with others of a like size and inclination than on the *content* of a particular play. Thus the lonely only child looks forward with delight to the *fact* of a party, and to the games that will be played at the party, and not to the games themselves, because the games are for him the expression of inclusion in a group. Just as an adult, looking after a solitary child during an afternoon, will say, " It played quietly ", and not specify the form of play, so a lonely child at a party will not differentiate sharply between game and game, or stress a delight in " Oranges and Lemons ", and object to " Blind Man's Buff "; love " Hunt the Slipper ", and dislike " Hunt the Thimble "; but will combine the series into a pleasurable whole.

This spontaneous pleasure in forming part of a group is not possible to the neurotic child. In place of an inner impulse to *share* enjoyment of this kind, the neurotic child has quite different feelings towards a group. To have a spontaneous impulse towards joining in a group, a child or a grown-up must feel in himself that he is *like* the members of that group.

A neurotic child either feels himself to be radically different from the other children of the group, or *is* in fact somewhat different. Feeling this, he lacks the primary essential for association with a group. He, therefore, fears hostile comment from other members of a group, and is in consequence unable to trust himself to them. Moreover, he knows himself to be possessed of feelings often and persistently of an anti-social type. He may, therefore, well be unable to join in a group, because he feels that if he were to attempt to join in at all, he would wish to fight, and not play, with the other members of the group.

The next quality which is essential for an enjoyment of group games is a certain

FLUIDITY OF EMOTION

Any group game, however simple, contains a continuous variety of emotional experiences for each child who takes part in it. Consider, for example, the child playing " Touch ". At one moment he is part of a group being chased—he feels himself a quarry chased by a hunter, and has all the emotions of the quarry. Then comes a sudden touch; he is caught, and, after a momentary feeling of being a captive, he becomes in his turn the hunter, with permission to enjoy the excitement of the chase. To play the game well and to enjoy the play, the child must rejoice in this change and interchange of emotions within the game. Indeed, the swiftly changing emotional attitudes which are characteristic of children have often bewildered adult observers. The funeral that begins as a sad memorial and ends as a joyous enterprise, and the party scene which begins cheerfully and ends in a " disaster " and " death ", cause dismay in the adult observer. Formerly such things were held to represent mere changeableness, a weakness of childish character that had to be eventually surmounted, and it was held that concentration was best induced by the imposition of long tasks of great monotony. During this century, however, this "changeableness" has been recognised instead as a fundamental phenomenon of youth and part of its characteristic quality. The adult attitude of censorship of this "fault" has changed to one of disinterested observation and of record without adverse comment. Otto Ernst[30] gives a charming example of this quality when describing a funeral played by his daughter Roswitha and some friends:

"But I must take a look at that funeral. It cannot be said that it seems a very doleful affair to them. On the contrary, they set to work as merrily as well-paid mourners. But before long there is a change—a change that I always made when I was a boy; they cease playing with dolls, and begin to play with human beings. Roswitha declares with great enthusiasm that she will be buried herself."

These changes are of the very nature of healthy childhood, and it is the desire to experience or express this very turmoil of emotion that lies at the root of much zest in group games. A child who is fixed in a certain attitude, always aggressive, always timid, always shy, etc., is totally unable to share in such games.

The following is an example from the I.C.P. records of incapacity to join in a group game:

G.D., Boy, aged 7. He was rather fascinated by the acting clothes, but fearful of accepting any rôles. He refused every part offered to him, such as bridegroom, father, priest, etc. Finally, when it came to a choice of being in the play or not, he said, "I want to be a silly thing, just nothing at all", and sat on the floor.

Here evidently, as he wished to be *in* the play (rather than be audience), there was a desire to join in, but he was unable to contemplate sharing the corporate emotion of the play, and so had eventually to put himself out of it.

Another quality which is necessary before any organised game can come into being is a

CAPACITY TO CONCEIVE FORM

One of the great difficulties encountered by healthily developing children in playing games with neurotic children, is the common failure of the latter group to grasp the necessity of form in a game. Unless there is a general acceptance of form of some kind, no type of social game, except rough and tumble movements and unorganised group games, can come into being. Many neurotics have such a riot of internal emotion that no continuity of form is possible to them.

Two little boys settling down to play, and deciding on "being" Nelson and Hardy and all the battle of Trafalgar, or two little girls deciding that they will dress a doll and live a day of her life, feel interfered with if they have to break off before they have completed their visualised scene. Nelson's death would terminate the one game, and the doll coming to bedtime would complete the other, each game having an outline to the children which is clear and definite. It is this capacity to see the series of movements necessary to complete a sequence as a whole which is the basic necessity for acceptance of the rules of social games.

A certain amount of emotional freedom is necessary before such a condition becomes possible. The child absorbed by inner problems and difficulties cannot achieve sufficient detachment to make this acceptance of rule possible. Here is an illustration:

E.C., Boy, aged 4. (At dancing.) I saw him sitting on the seat; he had refused to dance with the others. After some time I went to him and asked if he would sit on the floor with me and copy what the others were doing. He replied, " I must sit on the seat, I have *such* a lot to think about." At that moment dancing finished, and, on being told he could go, he dashed off his seat and to the door outside alone.

The neurotic child is at a double disadvantage. His emotions are not always conscious, and his will to pay attention is poorly practised and developed. A humorous example of this difficulty in conceiving the necessity of form in a game will be remembered by all who saw the skit on a Russian play produced by the late Sir Nigel Playfair, when the footballer comes home in his football clothes and replies to the question whether the game is over: " No, but suddenly, in the middle of the game, it came to me that there was no need for this striving, and I came away."

Parallel with the capacity to conceive form is the

CAPACITY TO KEEP A RULE

To keep a rule, even to one's personal disadvantage or to the disadvantage of one's side, entails a viewing of the game as a whole. The outlook of the person who takes a delight in the exact keeping and interpretation of rules of games is an objective one, and shows a keen interest in the interaction of individual against individual, or side against side.

It has been the viewpoint of the English race for a considerable period that the " play " or sport of their children should exercise those qualities that will be required later in the serious work of life. Thus, youths of the eleventh and twelfth centuries enjoyed taking part in tournaments and watching them as models of later conduct; and throughout the earlier centuries the sport of hawking and the hunting of dangerous animals have been considered " manly " and suitable " practice " for youths who might at any time be called upon to fight personally for the defence of an overlord or a king.

When, during the Victorian era, commerce began to be the main occupation of adult man in this country, such games as cultivated qualities that a man would be expected to need in the serious business of life came into prominence. Playful testing of moral qualities that would be needed later in adult work replaced playful training of man's muscle and nerve to the crucial occupation of fighting, and there was born a conception of the character-forming qualities of organised games—a conception that, although with diminished power, still holds the field to-day.

With this conception in the background, it is easy to see how it has arisen that to the adult the rules appear to be the essential characteristic of a game governed by rules, while to children these rules, and the learning of them, easily appear drudgery. It is the rules in a boxing match that prevent the opponents killing one another and turn the match into sport, but to the boy, excited and anxious to punch his opponent, the rules of boxing appear merely as an annoyance. A set of actions cannot become a " game " until the emotions that drive them have become sufficiently disciplined to be able to desire and accept a rule.

At the I.C.P. there are no instances of children's capacity to keep rules in group games, as no organised group games are played.

The normal child's natural tendency to cheat when it is small—or, rather, to remake the rules in its own favour or in the favour of a loved one, to fit what it views as special conditions—is watched anxiously by the careful parent or nurse, and carefully checked if it persists over nursery age. The normal English child is expected, by the time it reaches school age, to have learnt " group honesty " in its home and nursery play as much as it is expected to have learned personal honesty in regard to possessions. The child who fails to show this quality is a child who risks ultimate ostracism from his fellows. Nor must it, on the other hand, be forgotten that at a certain stage certain childen develop an aptitude for the invention of very strict and exacting rules of play for themselves. But this is not universal, and the origin of the desire is not yet clear.

The fifth necessity for enjoyment of a group play is a

Capacity to Subordinate One's Own Wishes to the Wishes of the Group

This capacity is essentially the basic quality upon which the previous capacity—that of keeping a rule—is founded. An ability to accept the wishes of the majority of a group as a guide to one's own behaviour is a sign that the first stages of civilisation, as we know it, have begun. Group games can assist, perhaps more than any other single factor, in helping a child to overcome his tendency to become fixed in one or other emotional condition. Temporary fixation in an emotional state, aggressiveness, jealousy, etc., cannot, unless it has reached a pathological condition, survive the joint gaiety and *élan* of a group's enjoyment of whatever activity it is prosecuting. A normal child who is temporarily cross or fretful will soon succumb to a group's enjoyment of a good group game; a passionate outburst and its exhausting after-effects will quickly be wiped out by participation in some jolly game of a group, and the experience gives the child a counterpoise to the oppressive power of his own emotions.

A further necessary quality is the

CAPACITY TO GET EMOTIONAL RELEASE OUT OF IDENTIFICATION WITH A GROUP

Emotional isolation is the characteristic of the neurotic, whether adult or child, and a capacity to identify oneself emotionally with a group is a capacity no neurotic can attain: he is inhibited by strong emotions, of whose presence he is only partly aware and whose nature he does not understand. The animation and emotion of the group form a swirling, dangerous sea around him, leaving him doubtful and fearful of being able even to attempt to swim in such unknown waters. If his emotional values are entirely individual, as they so often are, he cannot shout with a crowd with conviction: but from fear of being even more "different" if he remains silent, he will often do so in the end. His shouting, however, is not in direct response to a need to express an emotion shared by the others, but merely a mask to hide an inner difference. Thus he obtains no emotional release from his shouting as do the others, and in consequence is only frightened or bewildered or angered by what seems to him the "senselessness" of such group activity. As such exercise does not provide for him the emotional release it gives to the others, because inside himself he is forced to stand apart from them, it cannot appear to him anything but senseless. This contempt is then reciprocally felt, and he is resented as much by the group as he himself resents their actions.

Finally, there is necessary a

CAPACITY FOR LOVE OF ONE'S FELLOWS

Inhibition in object love is again a mark of a neurotic individual, and particularly so in the case of children. A neurotic individual is invariably mentally aware, at one level of consciousness or another, of his difference from his fellows. Love cannot travel spontaneously from individual to individual unless there are elements of likeness in the two individuals. As we have seen in Chapter II, where we considered sources of error in the mind, the mind cannot take in that which is totally unfamiliar to it. Conscious or unconscious difference, therefore, acts as a substantial barrier to object love between children. The child who grows up without the proper development of object love becomes inevitably an ego-centric individual, loving only himself. He cannot play in a group, because he cannot love any of the members of the group, although, if not in other ways inhibited, he may use the group to display his own superiority. For instance:

E.R., Boy, aged 13. In the rhythm room he was superior to the other boys in skill, but was rather slack, and showed an attitude of slight contempt towards the other. He sat in a corner and watched, now and then condescendingly doing an exercise to show his superiority.

The ego-centric individual may dominate over the group, and use it as a power instrument, or he may force the group into the expression of definite and dramatic phantasies of his own. But in these forms he is not joining in a group, and is hardly aware of the group at all—he is merely using it as he might use drawing or the figures of a " world " to represent a phantasy in his own mind. Games of this kind are considered in Chapter X.

CHAPTER IX

THE COMIC ELEMENT IN PLAY

*" Il semble que le comique ne puisse produire son ébranlement qu'à la condition de tomber sur une surface d'âme bien calme, bien unie. L'indifférence est son milieu naturel. Le rire n'a pas de plus grand ennemi que l'émotion."**

HENRI BERGSON.[44]

I T HAS BEEN SAID by E. R. Murray[45] that Froebel was without a sense of humour.** This is surprising to us in view of his creative work in education. But to-day we have a more liberal view of laughter than existed in England at the beginning of the century when Sully in his *Essay on Laughter*[46] apologises for, or excuses, his choice of this subject. Hearty laughter is no longer considered gross and undignified, but, on the contrary, it is accepted that it is often to be found associated with extreme courage—as, for example, in the case of Bairnsfather's Old Bill[47].

Hitherto very little study has been made of laughter in children. The laughter and tears of children appear to have appealed to the educationalist and the philosopher only because of their charming interchange of light and shadow. The purity of childish laughter and the apparent slightness of the causes of childish tragedy have often been subjects for pietic description and philosophic comment. But spontaneous laughter is a vital necessity to children's good health and normal development. In wise education opportunities for laughter should be given that will bring about a change from the hilarity of the infant tossed in his father's arms, to the intellectually developed appreciation of the comic of adult life.

Although little work has been hitherto done upon the comic sense of children, very many philosophers have at one time or another attempted to arrive at the reasons for the laughter of adults. Perhaps the most comprehensive of the published studies of laughter is that of J.Y.T. Greig.[48] For the most part the laughter of children has hitherto been regarded as

*" The comic appears only able to achieve its dynamic effect when it encounters a serene and untroubled spirit. Neutrality is its natural element—laughter has no greater enemy than emotion."
**" Enjoyment of the comic never, I think, makes its appearance at all. Froebel had many gifts, but the saving sense of humour does not appear to have been among them."

being of so irresponsible and bubbling a nature as to appear to arise more from physiological than from psychological origins, and it has hardly been thought worthy of serious study. There are elements, however, in the laughter of children an understanding of which is of profound importance in the general mental hygiene of childhood, and the neglect of which leads later to as serious consequences as neglect of any other single factor.

In thinking of humour in relationship to human beings, there are two aspects to keep simultaneously in mind: that of the individual who laughs, and of the object at which he laughs. Do all children laugh with equal readiness? Are there children who rarely laugh? And, if so, have we any information as to which children laugh and which do not? Are the same objects laughter-provoking to all children, or does their funniness vary with different children?

Although little attention has been paid to the comic sense of *children*, the infant's smile or laugh has been the subject of many investigations, a summary of which will be found in Chapter II of Greig's study.

Charlotte Bühler[26] gives the following fundamental stimuli to laughter in the first year of life, with photographs showing typical children in these situations:

	Age in Months.
	1 2 3 4 5 6 7 8 9 10 11 12
Social laughter	
Laughter at play or movement	
Laughter at bodily stimulus	
Laughter when a toy is offered	
Laughter at words	
Laughter at change of bodily position	
Laughter at "make believe" hiding	
Awakening with laughter	

Professor Bühler comments:

" The earliest is also here—what we shall call henceforth social laughter; viz. smiling at the look of another person, or at hearing a voice. Only much later laughter and smile appear on other occasions. According to observations made until now, laughter is primarily a social reaction."

On the question of the universality of laughter among infants—that is to say, as to whether all infants respond equally to these stimuli—Charlotte Bühler makes some interesting comments.

With her helpers she found that children react to a test, suggestive of an experiment carried out by Darwin with one of his children*, in three ways. The following description of the test is given:

" The observer puts a handkerchief over the child's face, holding it firm for a second, saying in a sing-song way, 'Where is the child?' Another second later he takes the handkerchief away, with the words, 'There it is.' This is repeated many times."

The reactions of the children to this test are described as follows:

" Some defend themselves gloomily, a few remain indifferent, some defend themselves laughing and wriggling, and some lie quite still smiling or laughing and wait for the game to be repeated."

The following table gives an interesting basis for further observation of types.

	Ages			
	0.6–0.8	0.9–0.11	1.0–1.5	1.6–1.11
Negative	50	30	10	10
Neutral	10	10	10	—
Positive				
Playful	30	30	40	20
Jesting	10	30	40	70
Total	100	100	100	100

It is common knowledge that the capacity to appreciate humour in adults varies considerably from person to person. Beyond this work of Bühler's already cited, the writer has not been able to find any other observations of

* " At one hundred and ten days one of Darwin's children ' was exceedingly amused by a pinafore being thrown over his face and then suddenly withdrawn; and so he was when I suddenly uncovered my own face and approached his ' " (see Greig[48]).

the variations in children of power to perceive and respond to the comic. It seems probable that we are here dealing with an inborn quality, but it is also probable that the subsequent history of the child has power to develop or inhibit an original capacity to appreciate humour. The relation of humour to emotional conflict has been well described by Bergson.[44]

To pass to the second question—that of the occasions which provoke laughter—it would seem that there are three general situations which in very small children give rise to laughter—bodily movement, at first of parts and then of the whole body; skin sensations of various kinds, prominent among them the tickling sensations; and early situations of physical pretence.

Now, with regard to these situations, it is crucial to an understanding of the causes of laughter in children to note that the bodily movements which produce such joy in the small child do so only when they *arise from a basis of security*.

The small child swung up and down upon his father's foot, thrown high in the air in its father's arms, or rolled over and over in a bed by a smiling mother, is an infant experiencing the excitement and delight of movement, *founded upon a basic situation of absolute security*. The solidity of the bed beneath him, or the strength of his father's arms, are his absolute guarantee against danger, and, once reassured on this point, he can give himself whole-heartedly to enjoyment of the excitement of movement.

Quoting Miss Shinn's little neice Ruth, Greig[48] gives the following example of this delight:

"'At three months old, she liked to be tossed in her father's arms, and during the fourth month became very fond of a frolic, and would crow and smile in high glee when she was tossed in the air, slid down one's knees, or otherwise tumbled about; the first true laughter I heard from her was over such a frolic in the last week of this month (one hundred and eighteenth day); and in the first six months this was almost the only cause of laughter . . . Thus on the one hundred and thirty-third day, seated on her mother's foot and danced up and down (held by the arms), she wore an expression of rapt delight, and whenever her mother stopped she would set up a little cry of desire . . . In the twenty-fourth week her father began another play that was very delightful to her—swinging or tossing her into her mother's arms, or mine, to be swung back into his; sometimes the three of us passed her thus from one to another. This excited great hilarity; she reached her arms from one to another and laughed aloud; and when the frolic was stopped and she was taken from the room, she set up a remonstrant whine.'"

This delight in passive enjoyment of movement in apparent security persists throughout life, and forms the *raison d'être* of all the toboggans, helter-skelters, and roundabouts of our fun fairs. The adolescent girl or emotionally primitive older woman, screaming and calling out with excited giggles and uproarious laughter on the roundabout is responding to the emotion which moved her first in her parents' arms, and this emotion has its origin in the same mechanism: violence, passivity, unexpectedness, speed, risk, all embroidered upon a background of a certainty of bodily safety.

Every human being is aware of the laughter-provoking effect of tickling, though individuals vary greatly in their susceptibility to this stimulus. Sully[46], in his *Essay on Laughter*, devoted twelve pages to a study of tickling. An interesting parallel can be traced between Bühler's description of the reaction of some of her very small children to the handkerchief over their heads and Sully's description of the reactions of a subject being tickled.

"There are two easily distinguishable groups of movements: (*a*) a number of protective or *defensive* reactions which are adapted to warding off or escaping from the attack of the tickling stimulus; (*b*) movements expressive of pleasure and rollicking enjoyment, from the smile up to uproarious and prolonged laughter."

In both cases the observers note an attempt at defence against the stimulus, accompanied at the same time by uproarious enjoyment of it.

In his summary Sully writes:

"We may perhaps sum up the special conditions of the laughter-process under tickling as follows: when a child is tickled he is thrown into an attitude of indefinite expectancy. He is expecting contact, but cannot be sure of the exact moment or of the locality. This element of uncertainty would in itself develop the attitude into one of uneasiness and apprehensiveness; and this happens save when the child is happy and disposed to take things lightly and as play."

This corresponds with the varieties of response, ranging from anxiety to enjoyment, shown by Bühler's infants.

In her work on teasing, Bühler[26] quotes Scupin and Herzfeld Preyer on the capacity of very young children for the initiation, or appreciation, of pretence situations, and shows that the essence of the joke lies in the fact that the situation which is found to exist is the reverse of that which is expected—that is to say, it is contrast which is the laughter-provoking stimulus.

Humour in adults is the sudden perception of an unsuspected relationship, which previously has not been apparent, between two otherwise unrelated or incongruous ideas or objects. In children the idea of incongruity in the form in which it is perceived in adult life does not occur; phantasy bridges the gulf. Absurdity—that is to say, incongruity—occurs to the child only in relation to its personal possessions that it knows extremely well. Thus, its own hat on the cat's head is funny, but the illustration of the wolf in the grandmother's bonnet is not funny, because the child's world is a magic, fairy-tale place, where such incongruities are the happy normal. To them there is nothing inherently impossible—a nobbly stick of wood with two tinsel stars on one nob, representing a king in an elaborate drama, is laughter-provoking or comic to the adult, because of the incongruity between the ideal of royalty, two spots of tinsel, and the nobs of a stick. To the child it is a perfectly adequate symbol of royalty.

In Bühler's examples of *Scherz* (jest) and *Komik* (comic), in which four pictures are shown to the children and their reactions noted, there appears a kind of enjoyment of incongruity which is the parent of the adult perception of humorous difference.

In these pictures there are shown:

1. Incongruous absurdities of size—a tiny horse drawing a huge waggon, a small child in huge shoes and hat, etc.

2. Animals and birds, a plant and a table, with human attributes.

3. A woman emptying a whole pail to wash a small child's hands.

4. A man in a tree sawing off the branch upon which he is sitting.

Now it should be noted that all these pictures are connected with familiar objects in the everyday life of the children. Their reactions are divided as follows:

Amusement at the pictures in general without the child being able to specify at what he is amused: 2 years old, 100 per cent; 3 years old, 70 per cent; 4 years old, 64 per cent; 5 years old, 20 per cent; 6 years old, 11 per cent; 7 years old, 7 per cent; 8 years old, 0 per cent.

Ability to specify what it was in the pictures that was amusing is, in inverse order to that of the previous group: 3 years old, 30 per cent; 4 years old, 36 per cent; 5 years old, 80 per cent; 6 years old, 89 per cent; 7 years old, 93 per cent; 8 years old, 100 per cent. That is to say that by eight years old the pleasure these children felt in the incongruities of the pictures was conscious.

Up to six years the conscious amusement felt was on the whole evenly divided between the humour of incongruity of size and that of personification. After six the latter predominated, and, by eight, pictures 3 and 4 equalled the other two in popularity.

There are certain characteristics of humour which are common to all forms, and certain which predominate in children's fun, and appeal to adults only when they find themselves in the position of inferior beings in the presence of superiors—that is, in a position analogous to that of children.

Let us consider these characteristics in turn.

Surprise is a basic element in all humour. A funny incident or the funny point of a story relies upon the existence of a slight and unemphasised pause, after which an unexpected *dénouement* startles the hearer into laughter. Without an element of the unexpected, laughter is impossible. But there are many forms this unexpectedness may take, and some are peculiar to children or childlike people:

THE IRRUPTION OF THE IRRATIONAL INTO THE RATIONAL

Children, as has been said many times, live in a world of magic, and forced transition from the magical world of phantasy to the rigid routine-ridden world of adult life presses hardly upon them. The sudden occurrence, therefore, of absurdity, the irruption of the irrational into the rational, is to them a constant source of delight.

Examples of this have already been given in the consideration of Professor Bühler's pictures, and others will be found scattered through this chapter.

THE JOY OF THE INSULT TO AUTHORITY

All children enjoy "taking off" their elders; situations in which the grown-up appears in a ridiculous or a humiliating light, and situations in which the child wins in competition with the adult, are an endless delight to them. This same delight, carried through to adult life, gives point to those comic pictures of the revolt of subordinates against authority, especially against pompous authority, that are a constant element in popular fun.

Every child is constantly aware that it is smaller, weaker, and less wise than the people among whom it lives, and, when it is sure of the possibility of doing so in reasonable safety, it relieves this pressure by creating real or phantasy situations in which the adult is at a disadvantage and the child triumphs. Examples:

G.W., Girl, aged 13. She became aggressive to Mr. X, saying that he was a queer creature, that his trousers had shrunk, and so on over various other points in his clothes, and she ended by dabbing red paint all over his hands.

On another occasion. "Let's play at school. I'll be the mistress," she said, and stood on a small chair. "You sit there. Now, copy exactly what I do." She then wrote several phrases which were immediately rubbed out, and scolded worker for not having done anything. Worker complained that as she rubbed everything out, it was difficult to put anything down. She laughed uproariously, and hugely enjoyed the joke.

On another occasion. She presented worker with a pair of cotton knickers, although she was to play a girl's part, and insisted that she put them on over her skirt. Then she added two coats and a large turban, and danced round her, saying, "You do look a freak."

A.M., Boy, and G.W., Girl, both aged 13. They were both being rather giggly, drawing on the wall, one giving a line and the other making it into some kind of drawing, the boy getting more and more wild. Finally worker drew a a small circle enclosed in a large circle, which was turned by A.M. into a figure of his headmaster, who was nicknamed "Grumpy".

THE SUDDEN ERUPTION OF A BODILY INTEREST

In the cultural training of children a great many primitive interests come under ban. It is the discovery of modern dynamic psychology that the energy with which these interests were invested when they first came to the forefront of the child's mind does not evaporate when these interests have been pushed out of consciousness. Underground in the mind this energy persists, and it comes to clothe with interest many activities and objects that are derivatives of the original idea. Through a process first perceived and described by Freud, emotional energy which was attached originally to very primitive interests, such as have been considered, for example, in Chapter IV, gradually moves from these to associated interests in other levels of the mind, till it can emerge in some activity which still symbolically represents the forbidden interest, but which now can meet with the approval of the whole personality.

This process, even under the best conditions, lags and halts in places where development does not go smoothly. At such points energy tends to bank up, and, if no outlet is given to it, it may show its presence by neurotic symptoms. To quote Bergson[44]:

" Il semble que le comique ne puisse produire son ébranlement qu'à la condition de tomber sur une surface d'âme bien calme, bien unie. L'indifférence est son milieu naturel. Le rire n'a pas de plus grand ennemi que l'émotion."

The emotionally disturbed child is not susceptible to normal laughter. Such laughter as is possible to a child of this kind, when it comes is more of the nature of an hysterical symptom or a nervous giggle. In the normal child, healthy uproarious *rücksichtslos* laughter explodes these banked-up pockets of energy and restores the emotional balance within the child once again.

It is clear that such laughter cannot occur except with the permission of the whole nature of the child. The least disapproval of one part of the child's self of the pleasure that could be taken in the joke by the other part of the child—for example, in bodily or sex incidents or jokes—inhibits the uprush of laughter and gives it a furtive and unpleasant twist. Laughter that belongs properly to this section is Falstaffian laughter, gusty, full-bodied, explosive, and is, in the main, laughter concerned with functions of the human body.

Such laughter is buffoonery, and belongs to the pantomimes of the older comedians, to Dan Leno and Herbert Campbell, and to Wheeler and

Wolsey, and Laurel and Hardy of to-day. To a very cultivated adult, humour of this kind often borders on the disgusting, though to the uncultivated it performs, as in childhood, an exceedingly useful function. In the performances of these comedians the elements of insult to authority, licence in regard to bodily interests, and the irruption of the irrational into the rational are usually combined. Together they make up:

Buffoonery and Clowning

It is interesting to note that buffoonery and clowning, which in one form or another were at one time a constant element of the theatre and the circus, and were a common accompaniment of public holidays, have now sensibly declined. Hampstead Heath has become " civilised ", and even costers and the costers' parade have become as decorous as mutes.

The loss is a serious one for children.

Buffoonery is the explosion into action of emotions that find themselves under too great tension, and we are always apt to forget the strength of the emotions of childhood, and the necessity for relief.

Buffoonery is an essential element of good education. To be able to enjoy the unexpected, to perceive the incongruous, and to welcome the grotesque, is to start out with a good equipment to make sense of so strange a world as ours.

A good laugh, a piece of good-humoured horseplay at the right moment, the combination of a desire to tease, an impulse of affection and a burst of animal spirits into a physical joke, which is good-humouredly received, discharges an overplus of energy which otherwise can only too easily hamper serious intellectual work.

On the other hand, buffoonery can easily degenerate into an escape from work. The boy or girl who has learned to make his fellows laugh, and to win popularity thereby, tends to find the warmth that results so precious that he is in danger of adopting a burlesque attitude as his key to popularity, and his standard reaction to life.

Now, buffoonery can take many forms: for example, the making of oneself absurd; the decorating of one's face; the adding of a mask, a long nose, or a clown's colouring to one's own face. The chief exponent of this form of buffoonery is, of course, the clown in the circus, always beloved and often imitated by children.

Such imitation is associated with two desires: impersonation of the clown whom the whole circus has laughed at and loved, and the child's desire to be, like the clown, a " silly thing ".

This is a healthy impulse. To be able to enjoy the irrational, instead of being irritated by it, is a passport to life. Children and grown-ups who have laughed together do not easily fall out; laughter is the great healer of sores.

Another form of buffoonery is the making of someone else absurd. Some examples of this have already been given—here are some others showing the use of playroom material to this end.

M.E., Girl, aged 13. With mosaics she made a little man without a head, and said he was a " toffee-nosed orphan ". When she had finished the figure, she told Dr. L. that it was her.

G.W., Girl, aged 13. She made a grotesque figure in plasticine which was finally called a woman (though it was not made with the idea of being either sex). It was naked but for a hat (pudding basin), heavily trimmed, on top. A very large nose and lips were stuck on the face and practically obliterated it, and a piece of bread and butter was put in the mouth. The figure had very small arms and legs, but an enormously thick and long tail. Next G.W. made a man, equally grotesque, but with very long arms and legs, but no tail. She giggled a good deal throughout, and thoroughly enjoyed what she was doing.

Practical joking is another form of this love for making other people absurd. Its persistence in some cases in after-life was illustrated in the person of the late Sir Gerald du Maurier[49]. Here is a boyish example:

B.I., Boy, aged 9. He seized big bricks and built a sort of chair. He sat on it and it collapsed. He was very anxious to rebuild it and to get Dr. L. to sit on it. He did so, putting a duster and rug over so that it should look safe. When Dr. L. arrived, he said they must have a ceremony of enthroning her on a throne made by him, and M.S. must crown her. He was very excited, and laughed uproariously when Dr. L. sat on the throne and it gave way.

A clown is a person one laughs *at*—to love anyone properly one must be able to laugh at him a little. Every spontaneous child aches at some time or another to put the adult he loves to the test of seeing whether he be willing to be put into the clown's rôle at times, allowing the child to dominate, and himself appearing foolish. It eases the strain of the child's perpetual subordination to authority and redresses the balance of superiority. " Ragging " at the right place and in moderation is a valuable and healthy outlet for feelings of amusement at the adult which might easily turn into spite. For example:

M.E., Girl, aged 13. Her manner seemed quite natural and friendly until the close of the session, when she and another girl had a glorious " rag " for about ten minutes, both taking keen delight in dabbing wet and floury fingers on to everyone, children and adults alike, who came within arms' length.

On other occasion. She did a " bunny race ", rushing all over the playrooms, shouting at the top of her voice and laughing noisily. She climbed fearlessly over obstacles, then took to dancing and playing ball, but did all in a comic and rowdy manner.

B.G., Boy, aged 10. While talking to worker about football, he gave a full and dramatic description of the play of various halves, backs, and goalkeeper. The description of the hefty back of one team receiving and disposing of attackers with a contemptuous flick of his hip was convulsingly funny and extraordinarily well done.

Buffoonery can also be expressed by the imagining of playing out absurd re-creations and elaborations of actual scenes.

Here comes in all humanity's delight in the banana peel, and the eternal joy of Chaplin, and of the standard long and short music-hall couples. The pleasure in them is shared by adults and by children, and is the kind of pleasure that makes the appeal of those comic papers so much beloved by children.

Herein also lies the source of the "cruelty" of children and of primitive people. To the child the burst boiler, the motor-lorry in the shop window, and to the primitive person the writhings of a victim under verbal or physical torture, tend to provoke laughter rather than sympathy. It is impossible for them imaginatively to re-create, and so realise, the pain underlying the catastrophe. Understanding can be brought only by experience, and it is exactly this factor of experience that is lacking. Looked at externally, the positions resulting from these catastrophes *are* bizarre and odd, and oddness always tends to provoke laughter. Here are examples of played-out "cruel" scenes:

A.M., Boy, aged 12. He selected from the "world" tray the sitting figure of a woman and placed her on the side of the swimming-bath. He made her fall in frequently, and laughed heartily each time.

E.R., Boy, aged 13. He was playing with dolls, and made one dance about and stagger. It was said to be drunk. He then picked up the big rag doll, said it was the mother, and she was also drunk. During the whole time there was a broad smile on his face.*

On the same lines people tend to mock at the differences shown by other individuals or other groups than their own, or by odd-looking people *in* their group. Here arises the tragedy of the fat boy and the red-haired girl. Even the Institute is not free from such tendencies, as these examples show:

*During the discussion following this lecture a member of the audience quoted as an example of laughter at catastrophes a child in her school who made cemeteries with bricks. When asked whom he buried, he replied his relatives, and laughed inordinately at this.

K.T., Boy, aged 8. He was distinctly aggressive on the way down to the hall to play charades, and deliberately mimicked another boy's lame leg and awkward gait. This was again noticeable when doing free movement to music in the games. He followed the lame child closely round the room, grotesquing his movements very cleverly.

M.C., Girl, aged 12. She did some painting and then made dough. She giggled and fooled about, and sneered at another girl aged 11 for dropping an " h ".

Following upon buffoonery, of which all the above are examples, the second way in which the comic impulses of children tend freely to express themselves is in

CARICATURE

And caricature itself may have several forms; it may, for instance, be a simple blurring of features without any reference to the real nature of the actual individual represented.

This type of caricature is clowning narrowed down to a particular individual. The change brought about is usually an addition, and the features added are the standard symbols of comedy. The humour lies in the *lack* of appropriateness of the addition to the original face.

Where the clown is an impersonal figure and clowning has no relation to persons, caricature is an underlining of a particular concept concerning an individual. Clowning is uproarious and good-tempered; caricature has always a faintly malicious intent.

The red nose of a drunkard, signifying drink and not good humour, moustaches and whiskers attached to a female face, the long pointed nose and claw fingers of a witch, the big ears of the fool, the traditional pointed cap of the dunce, the big teeth of the so-called wolf, are the usual features which tend to be added to the portrait in this most primitive form of caricature. The procedure is to make the face or figure by drawing or modelling or representation in any material that is suitable, and with shouts of laughter to add one or other of the traditional features.

The humorous idea in this case is the suggestion that the benevolent or reverend figure represented might *in reality* possess the added characteristics if one only knew.

M.E., Girl, aged 12½. She drew on the board " portraits " of several of the workers and one of the other children. All the drawings had very long noses. In the case of Mr. X, she prolonged the nose to grotesque dimensions, and said, " I would like to put some drips on the end of his nose, but the board is not big enough." Most figures, particularly the ones of female workers, had spikes projecting between the legs. One had a head with a great many teeth and very much exaggerated eyes. One child and Miss Y were drawn as pigs.

G.W., Girl, aged 13. She drew portraits of another girl and two workers. They were very crude and infantile for a girl of 13, and their chief feature was a mouth spreading from ear to ear filled with enormous teeth. On another occasion she again drew people, the chief features this time being hair standing straight up like wire.

This exaggeration may be of actually existing characteristics, with a spiteful undercurrent.

When children take to this form of caricature, only the most superficial characteristics of the individual are chosen. Few children have sufficient insight into the characters of adults or of their own playmates to see the traits lying beneath the surface.

Caricatures at the I.C.P. are carried out in pencil, paint, or modelling, or can be expressed in the mimicry of acting (see section dealing with mimicry). For example, the writer herself has a bumpy nose, and a small girl represented this as under:

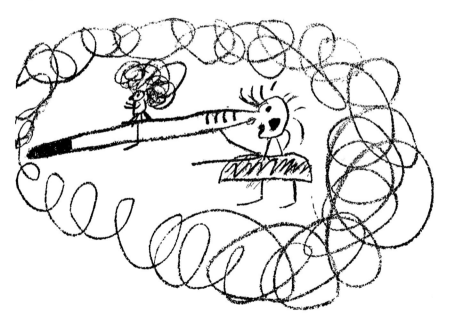

Another male worker, himself actually of a kindly disposition, had come to stand to a boy of thirteen for a master he particularly disliked and

dreaded. With a sudden inspiraton one day he seized a soft pencil and drew
the drawing given below:

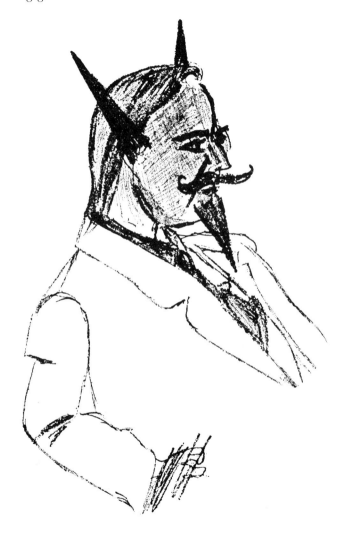

This picture incorporates the characteristic features of Mephistopheles
with a fair approach to a likeness of the boy's model. The rest of the paper
was covered with insulting and deprecatory epithets applied to this and all
the other adults in the room. The boy's emotional tension was sensibly
diminished by the creation of this drawing.

Children are sometimes unable to see an individual at all for the fog of emotion that the individual arouses in them. This is to a certain extent true of all emotionally disturbed children, but when to this feeling is added an urge for expression and an interest in a pencil point, amusingly fantastic drawings result. The creation of these figures gives the children great satisfaction, and from them considerable insight can be gained into the forces at work in the child's mind. These representations, as the above shows, are often quite fantastic, and their humour lies in a combination between malice and absurdity.

The difficulty with so many children is that their degree of technical skill is not sufficient to allow them outlets of this kind, and it is here that the "grotesques" (see p. 30) come in so usefully. Various firms of toy manufacturers make collections of painted pieces of wood or composition cut in various shapes which allow of the composing of grotesque and absurd figures. For the child who would love to make caricatures but has not the necessary technical skill these sets of pieces form a very valuable outlet.

Children use these in various ways. Sometimes they make a series of pigmies and christen them with the workers' names or the names of their teachers or members of their family; sometimes to give the child release it suffices for him to create neutral figures of utter absurdity without otherwise personifying them. Sometimes traditional figures are made such as Humpty Dumpty or Little Bo Peep with grotesque additions.

Whole scenes are sometimes invented to give vent to children's hidden emotions.

Many children feel very bitterly about their schools or their environment, and some children can work off this feeling by writing plays which consciously "take off" troublesome elements in their lives.

The following are two plays dictated to the writer with shouts of laughter by a boy of nine, much in trouble with authority, and were written down as dictated.

A FUNNY PLAY

CHARACTERS

A. A fat, red-nosed man. Workman.
B. A very lanky policeman with red face.
C. A fat and bustling old woman.
D. A very posh spick-and-span man. Fat.
E. A lanky sweep.
F. A very solemn parson.
G. A very solid, slow, bad-tempered policeman.
H. A labourer.
L. A wooer.
M. A shopman.

(The first five were set out before the play began and the others added one by one as they occurred to him.)

ACT I

SCENE I

A policeman holding up traffic and ordering people to stop, and a very little car comes along (very rickety) and hits him in the tummy with a very sharp front. Cuts him right in two and goes on.

SCENE II

At the next stop a very posh, spick-and-span man, fat, is crossing the road. He gets bumped into the back of a car, which shoots him right up into the air. He says, "Oh, you little beast—my bottom. I've got my Sunday-go-to-meeting trousers on!" He tumbles down a chimney where a lanky sweep is sweeping, and hits his broom with his head. D says, "Oh, my head." He hits the sweep on his nose and gives him a huge swelling on it. The sweep is dazed and cries, "Why, what's this? My blasted nose." Mr. Tubby gets stuck in the chimney and yells and yells, and eats tomatoes which he has in his pocket; one is squashed much too much to make it eatable.

SCENE III

So he chucks this tomato out of the top of the chimney and it hits the bustling fat old woman on her head and lands right in a basket of eggs, and hits the eggs, because it was a funny tomato with a stone inside. "Oh, lawks!" says she. The eggs split and squash and splash up into her face and that of a fat, red-nosed workman, and of a very solemn parson who gets very angry and so red. The policeman sees, picks a beetroot out of the woman's basket (a very soft one), and chucks it at the clergyman full in the face. He goes flop, and comes up again with fury and picks up a baby in a passing pram and chucks it at the policeman. The policeman dodges, and the baby goes flying on and down the chimney and hits Mr. Tubby's pocket full of tomatoes, and both go down the chimney together and fall flop into a large saucepan, and the old lady thinks they are pork and boils them for dinner—and says: "Ah, what a nice present somebody has sent me."

ACT II

SCENE I

The sweep meanwhile goes home with the bump on his nose. His wife says: "Darling, what has happened to you?" The sweep says: "Why, something tumbled down the chimney and hit me full on the nose." His wife says: "I'll bandage it up for you, dear, and I'll put you to bed." Which she does.

SCENE II

The fat red-nosed man who had the tomatoes in his face goes home blubbing, and his wife is so angry with him for spoiling the cap he had just bought for 1s. 4d., because they were so poor, she chucked him into the mill-pond, where he was drowned.

SCENE III

The parson, who was just going to preach, says: " I can't preach like this." " Why not, mister? Liven us up a bit," says a labourer. The parson gets very angry and hits the labourer, and the policeman takes them both up and knocks their heads together and takes them to jail, where they are executed next day.

SCENE IV

Meanwhile the old woman went weeping on her way home. She was met by her young lover, who said: " Dear, darling, what is the matter with you?—and she blubs out: " My eggs are all smashed and we won't have anything to eat for lunch." " Oh, well, dear, don't mind; we can go and get some tiddly-widdlies from the sweet counter." " Right you are", says the old woman, and when she gets to the thing she says to the shopman: " Can I have two pounds of tiddly-widdlies?" He is a very quick-tempered shopman, and takes up a pound of sticky toffees and chucks them right in her face. She tries to scratch these off her face and scratches her eyes out. The shopman chucks all the stuff in the shop at her face, and she yells and screams till she is dead.

FINISH

SECOND PLAY

Programme 1d.
CHARACTERS
Mrs. Silly Owl.
Mr. Silly Owl.
Mincing Mary.
Boastful Bill.
Jumping Jack.
Quarrelling Jane.
Mr. Googley.

ACT I

Scene I . . . . The dining-room at breakfast time.

ACT II

ACT I
SCENE I

The table is laid for breakfast. There are four chairs and two steps at the back of the room. There is a teapot with water in it, and remains of a banana on the floor.

Mr. Silly Owl, coming downstairs in a hurry, slips on the banana skin and bumps into Jumping Jack and upsets him. "Oh, blast!" says he. "Who left that there? Yaow!" Jack doesn't mind, as he bounces up and down and hits Mincing Mary on her way to breakfast. Mary tries to hit back and hits her dad instead, and he is very angry. "You horrible girl—you get worse every day. To-day you shall eat your breakfast under the table."

Mrs. Silly Owl comes downstairs dolefully and weeps into the cream jug, upsetting it over the table and everybody's legs.

Mr. Silly Owl: "Oh, dear. How can I go to the City like this?"

Quarrelling Jane: "You look such an ass, anyway, we don't think anyone will notice the difference."

Mrs. Silly Owl, weeping: "I wish you were not so rude to your dad, Jane. You always quarrel with everyone. No one helps me."

Exit Mr. Silly Owl.

Jumping Jack, jumping up to punish Jane, upsets the breakfast-table, and everyone is in a muddle in the table-cloth on the floor. Mrs. Silly Owl runs round with her handkerchief trying to get them all straight and making the muddle worse all the time.

Mincing Mary emerges with a pat of butter on her nose, which she doesn't notice, and says mincingly, "Oh, dear, mother, these children are very rude. Why are you weeping, mother dear?"

Boastful Bill: "*I* know—I know everything. I know why mother weeps."

Quarrelling Jane pushes him out from under the table.

"Oh, you always think you know everything. You probably know why Mary has a pat of butter on her nose."

Mary claps her hands to her nose and brings them away smeared with butter, and bursts into tears, while Jack solemnly pours the teapot over her. She retires to the background, where she and her mother weep together. Jane pummels Bill for having made her cry.

Boastful Bill: "Now, children, be quiet. I will tell you the reason of all this trouble." (Puffs out his chest.)

Jumping Jack: "Shut up, you idiot."

Boastful Bill (goes on): "All this trouble in a peaceful, in a beautiful spring morning is really deplorable."

Jumping Jack shuts him up with a cushion.

Mrs. Silly Owl (puts away her handkerchief): "I am afraid I am the cause of all this trouble. You see, I found a black banana, and I liked it so much I had to leave a piece of it on the floor for your dear dad to see, but he slipped on it instead and then all this trouble came—I am a most unfortunate woman."

All at once: "No, mummie, you are very nice—we like you very much. Please be cheerful." They surround her, and all walk out of the room.

SCENE II

The master's desk with books on it. Two children's desks with inkpots (full of water). A door.

Made to stay in: Boastful Bill.
　　　　　　　　Jumping Jack.
　　　　　　　　Teacher (male).

Boastful Bill finishes what he had got to do and starts off: "You see, my brother, how clever I am. I have added 2 to 2 in half an hour and got it quite right. Look, I have looked at the answer—isn't it wonderful? You couldn't do that."

Jumping Jack is very cross and picks up teacher's inkpot and throws it right at Boastful Bill. Boastful Bill dodges just as teacher comes into the room, and it catches him full in the chest and spills all down him.

Boastful Bill gets frightened and runs away.

Jumping Jack quickly gets on to work, and teacher, turning round, seeing Boastful Bill running away, thought that it was him, and goes after him with a cane. Boastful Bill is too quick.

Jumping Jack gets into teacher's coat and hat, and sits in his seat.

Mincing Mary, very full of her clothes, etc., comes mincing in to ask when the boys are coming home, and sees what she thinks is teacher sitting at the desk.

Mincing Mary: "Oh, Mr. Googley, mother wants to know when the boys are coming home because their dinner is getting cold."

Jumping Jack (in high voice): "Well, you know, I had no sausages for my dinner, so I boiled both those boys and ate them. Would you tell their mother, please, they are my dinner, so they won't come home for dinner."

Mincing Mary runs away with a scream.

Jumping Jack tears his coat off and jumps round the room.

Mr. Googley returns (still with black face) and Jumping Jack, shrieking with laughter, says, "I've just told Mary that you've eaten us for dinner. Ha! ha! ha!"

Mr. Googley is overcome with horror and sinks into a chair and mops his face.

ACT II

Going to bed. Children's room. Three beds. The children come in together—peaceful.

Jumping Jack: "Let's have a pillow fight."

Boastful Bill: "Yes, I'm awfully good at pillow fighting."

Mincing Mary: "No, it's too rough."

Quarrelling Jane: "How like you, Mary, not to fall in with anything we want to do."

Mincing Mary: "I don't like to get myself dirty and my hair rumpled like boys do."

The two boys have started already, and Boastful Bill gets a huge whack on the head from Jack. Mincing Mary tries to separate them daintily and elegantly, but Quarrelling Jane pulls her away and joins in. . . General scrimmage.

The door opens and Mrs. Silly Owl walks in and says: "Oh, my poor pillows. Lie down at once, you children. Oh, why can't you stop quarrelling? Oh, do lie down."

The children put down the pillows and, sighing to each other, all three lie down wrong way up, with their toes on the pillow, except Mincing Mary, who smugly lies the right way. Mrs. Silly Owl does not notice and walks slowly out of the room weeping.

THE END

It is amusing to note in plays of this kind the occasional intrusion of words or phrases remembered from grown-up conversation.

Passing from caricature, which has always a human content, we come to

WIT

Real wit is an adult accomplishment, but childish wit includes puns, riddles, and rhymes, nonsense rhymes, and the fun of verbal malapropisms. Wit appeals to very few children, but there is an age when puns and riddles are of absorbing interest, and the child spends his day trying every riddle he knows upon everyone he meets, and doing his best to make up new versions of his own. Here are instances from the Institute records:

M.C., Girl, aged 11. A rowdy and exhibitionist spirit broke out in her. She made silly puns about the sewing materials, laughing uproariously herself, and enjoying another girl's hysterical appreciation of her jokes.

A.J., Girl, aged 6. While in the shop, she said to worker, " You be gold man."
Worker: " What is a gold man?" A.J.: " A gold man is a man who makes
gold." (Laughter.)

A.J., Boy, aged 7. A scene is set out on a table: a garage and two lamp-posts
placed beside it. A lorry drives into one. A policeman comes up and says,
" What is your number?"
Driver: " Cucumber!"
Policeman: " How dare you? What's your number?"
Driver: " Black Man Cumber."
Policeman: " Take a black eye." Gives him one.

This rather obscure witticism rejoiced the whole roomful of children.

M.B., Girl, aged 7. She drew pictures which were riddles for the worker to
guess, as follows:

1. Find ball lost in rose-garden.
2. Find end of tangle (circular lines drawn as in maze).
3 and 4. Finding balls in field.

The next four baffled the worker, but looked like:

5. Boats with two sails.
6. A house with two chimneys.
7. A lighted candle.
8. A figure wearing dunce's cap.

9 and 10 were guessed correctly as a face and a showman.

G.W., Girl, aged 13. She showed me many rhymes made up by herself,
concerned with a master, Mr. Innocent. The conception was very poor
and the general level very childish, but it aroused excited giggles in her.

On another occasion. She picked up a chalk and spontaneously wrote on the
wall:

> " *Old farmer Buck, he bought him a duck,*
> *And he cut off her feet, 'cos she walked in the muck.*
> *And when she wouldn't go for to roost like a crow,*
> *He cut off her feet for to make him so.*"*

HUMOUR

Humour, which is the perception of an unexpected, and at the same time
amusing or curious, aspect of common happenings, by its very nature

---

*During the discussion following this lecture a member of the audience quoted that one child
related, " We had roast beef and potatoes and greens." Another child squashed this by saying,
" We had roast beef and potatoes and greens and yellows."

cannot occur in children. In adults, fashion and trend of thought change so quickly that concepts of the humorous are notoriously unstable. One generation wonders at the humorous stories which in another generation provoked loud laughter.

NONSENSE

With nonsense it is a different story. Several North European nations show a delight in nonsense. It may be that this delight is a special variation of the general rule concerning the irruption of the irrational into the rational as if one would say, "Among so much sensible use of words, a *nonsensical* use is delightful." Humorous children have a never-ending delight in this kind of fun. "Goose, boose, hoose, toos", chanted a friend of mine of seven, for the plural of "horse" is "heese", and "a boose boose goose is toos." The irrational is a relief from the rational, and nonsense enjoyed for a while leaves the mind fresher for sense.

Stanley Hall[13] quotes an example of this:

"'I never saw a hawk, but I can hawk and spit too.' 'I will not sing do re mi, but do re you.'"

Continental conceptions of this form of fun differ. Nonsense in German is reiteration of incompatible facts in rhyme. Nonsense in French is a definite "baby section", split off from ordinary language as we split off "baby talk", and the French elaborate the comic for children until the Christmas shop decorations are so mechanical that children are awestruck at what should amuse them. Nonsense in England may as often as not be created by, and enjoyed by, intellectual adults; *vide* "The Jabberwock" by the mathematician Dodgson (Lewis Carroll).

The never-failing popularity of the limerick, of collections of schoolboy howlers, of Christmas-book nonsense rhymes, historical parodies, and comic verse, shows how popular this form of enjoyment of the ridiculous is among people of all ages in this country.

MIMICRY

In *An Essay on Laughter*, Sully[46] writes of the urge to imitate:

"The attitude of reverence towards superiors has for its psychological concomitant the impulse to imitate. Just as children will copy the voice and gestures of one whom they look up to, so savages will copy the ways of Europeans who manage to make themselves respected."

In the same way as there is an impulse in all children towards imitation of their elders, particularly of elders who are liked and admired, so in some children there is an irresistible impulse to "take off" a prominent elder. To "take off" another person one feels oneself into the character by empathy and observation, and then expresses an impulse to mock at, belittle, or humiliate the adult by giving a twist to our representation of him. These are examples:

A.J., Girl, aged 6. She did a drawing of a boy and fixed it on the wall with a bit of plasticine. She then found a man's hat, put it on, and did a comic dance of the chorus-girl type, which she hugely enjoyed. She then invented a game in which she impersonated several sorts of characters very well. This child is a born mimic and seems to get emotional release in acting the comic.

E.R., Boy, aged 13. He hated the suggestion of playing school with some other children, but when it was changed to the idea that he should be schoolmaster, he stood up and put his fingers in the armholes of his waistcoat in a most amusing pantomime of a pompous and imposing master.

J.D., Girl, aged 6. She was aware of her surroundings all the time, and interested in two boys. She ignored a girl who insisted upon playing with her. She mimicked unkindly another girl's rather insistent little voice, and got a good deal of pleasure out of the mimicry.

Two remaining forms of laughter have to be considered: giggling and the use of the comic directly to express animosity.

GIGGLING

Giggling can arise from many sources.

(*a*) Nervousness. A child who feels uncertain of his reception by a group, and wishes very much to be accepted, but is uncertain of his capacity to produce the right impression, gives vent to the complexity of this emotion by giggling. For example:

M.C., Girl, aged 12. She was shy and monosyllabic at first, but with a little encouragement agreed to express rhythms in movement, but never really let herself go. She made dough, but did not do anything definite; just giggled and fooled about. It was difficult to get her to do anything with the dough, to go home at the end of the session, or to leave the dough behind.

On another occasion. She came down to dancing with another girl and did absolutely nothing. She giggled from start to finish and was very unlike the painstaking child I had had before.

(*b*) Delight in sharing a slightly improper joke, or in suddenly perceiving something slightly improper in a situation.

(c) The excitement of effort which is unexpectedly unsuccessful produces a kind of physical nervousness which often has an outlet in giggling.

THE COMIC AS AN EXPRESSION OF ANIMOSITY

There is a little opportunity in a social community for the permissive expression of animosity, and conscious animosity, if it is not expressed, tends to bank up dangerously within the individual. The comic provides a way out of this difficulty.

With younger children a sense of the comic is apt to take the form of rudeness, and this rudeness, though appearing to an adult merely rude, strikes the child himself, and the children who hear it, as uproariously funny. With older children this impulse is more often expressed in caricature, or the christening of an adult or other child with an amusing nickname whose appropriateness arises out of spiteful observation. Examples:

M.E., Girl, aged 13½. As she could not get the attention of Dr. L., who was working with another child, she continually tried to do so by making insulting and ribald remarks, some of them personal remarks, about Dr. L.'s appearance, many of a rather spiteful kind, and some frankly funny.

J.B., Boy, aged 6. On being asked if he was going to give his brother a birthday present, he said he was going to give him a "clout round the head".

P.T., Boy, aged 4. He ran and put some sand in an older boy's clean water when he wasn't looking, then laughed mischievously.

In a setting such as the I.C.P., occasions for expressions of this kind are rare, since the children develop the type of relationship to the workers and to each other in which such incidents do not readily grow.

It is, however, possible to point out to children who are much troubled with hostile feelings that expression of a spiteful thought can often be tolerated if given a humorous twist, and that learning at the same time to take a laugh against oneself makes one invulnerable against spiteful attacks. Not to be able to take a jest directed against oneself indicates a lack of that sense of security in a child upon which the enjoyment of all forms of humour depends.

"*Le rire n'a pas de plus grand ennemi que l'émotion*", says Bergson[44], and gives expression to a truth of profound value. Emotional conflict is the inhibitor of laughter, of all laughter that is not the laughter of malice and revenge. Only from a background of security can lovely laughter come. Laughter is the great healer, as it is the peacemaker among peoples, and when it is not malicious it is both the creator and the outer evidence of sanity.

CHAPTER X
CHILDREN WHO CANNOT PLAY

W E H A V E now considered the main classes into which children's play can be grouped, and are faced by a new problem: what is the relationship between the child himself and the forms his play takes? What impulses guide a child in the choice of a type of play, and why is it that some children appear to be unable to play at all?

If, from this new angle, we review the material we have collected, it will be seen that it can be analysd into three groups:

1. Play which is entirely isolated and personal and which needs for its performance only the most shapeless of materials.

2. Play which is still individual, but which creates out of the material it uses a definite objective play world with which it associates itself.

3. Playing out with fellow-players themes mutually agreed upon.

Day-dreaming is the extreme form of the first type of play. Theodate L. Smith[50] has made an interesting study of day-dreaming, and gives a good bibliography, at the end of his paper, of books and papers that refer to it. The next variety of Group 1 is the type of play illustrated by E.C. in Chapter V, page 112. He needed water and a tray to express the impulse that drove him to play, but the character and meaning they took was moulded entirely by the child's own thought. When asked to join a group of children moving about and doing something corporate, E.C. refused to do so, because he said, " I must sit on the seat, I have *such* a lot to think about " (see p. 173). Children whose play falls into Group 1 are children who have such a rich interior life of their own that they are unable to join with other children until they have had opportunity first to work out their own ideas. Group 1 is particularly the play of the very young child, or of the child who alternates play in a group with the working out of his own thoughts in play.

In Chapter V of this book will be found abundant instances of the second form of play, and they can be compared with those to be found in Stanley Hall and Ellis's study of dolls[13]. This is the play of the isolated child, whether it be isolated by physical fact or dominated by a type of phantasy which needs elaborate material for its working out, and which thus does not permit of the player combining with other children.

Group 3 represents the normal form of play of children from eight to ten years of age in those hours of the day when they are with other children. A healthy, imaginative child with adequate opportunity will in its total play hours of a week move successively through all these forms of play. But there are other aspects from which play may usefully be regarded. For example, the actual play may be shapeless, or may be run into the mould of form.

For example, here are instances of shapeless play.

C.B., Boy, aged 11. On arrival he had no idea of what he wanted to do, but ran round the garden aimlessly, kicking objects, hacking at branches and plants with his pocket-knife, which he keeps in a Buffalo-Bill sheath attached to his belt.

M.E., Girl, aged 10. She was rather listless, said she was going to work, and several times pointed out to people that she was working, but in fact she did scarcely anything. She asked frequently for another girl, but, when the other girl came, M.E. whispered to worker that she did not want her. M.E. chose plasticine, and made a head and a hat of a snowman, but the body was never finished. She then said she would make a village of snowmen, and put down on a tray some sand, two houses, and one man in front, then a ring of people who were supposed to be making a snowman, but she never gave her mind to the game. She vaguely wanted things that other people had, and at last took cardboard dolls and fitted them with paper dresses for no apparent reason. At the end of the afternoon she hung about till very late, making an attempt to tidy the room.

M.C., Girl, aged 12. She dressed up as a bride and showed off a little as such, then she changed to a princess, and readily fell into the rôle and desired a husband. She then suggested dancing as a finish, and danced with clumsy, ugly, violent gestures, saying she was a ballet-girl, but looked more like a football player. She laughed, looked self-conscious, and finally fell in making a big kick. Her movements were unco-ordinated and uncontrolled, and there was no shape or conception in the dance.

K.T., Boy, aged 7. He started throwing plasticine on the wall and hammering it, but was very unsettled, and then tried carpentry. He wanted to make a boat, and found sawing too hard work, so gave up the idea and went back to plasticine. Then he spied some water toys and water, and played with them, his chief occupation being pouring from one pot to another. He wanted some sand as well, but settled to nothing.

Instances in the section on noise in Chapter III, page 43, already given, are also examples of such shapeless play. What is it, then, that determines that play shall take any shape?

Some children, like the little boy quoted in Chapter V, page 112, or the little girl in Chapter IV, pages 103–104, once they have devised a form of play, show the most extreme reluctance to leave it. Such children ask again and again for the same story, and insist that each repetition shall be identical. Many children, on the other hand, are referred to the Institute for *lack* of concentration, for an inability to conceive any kind of form, and these children show themselves resistant to all attempts to help them to put either play or work into definite shape.

These two types certainly illustrate extreme cases, but they reveal a difference of temperament that runs right through the domain of child life. Recognition of such difference is a very real assistance to the observer who is trying to understand the play life of any group of children.

Play in children, as we have said, is the expression in action of ideas which are already present in the mind. If, then, a child's play is understood, a conception can conversely be gained from it of the nature of the ideas at work in the child's mind.

But between child and child there is a very wide variation in the fertility of this idea life of the mind.

We are all aware of the fact that different individuals vary greatly in the wealth of their ideas. Some children, as some grown-ups, are possessed with a rich flow of ideas, remember experiences well, and have the impulse to recombine experiences. Other children, without being necessarily deficient in intelligence, perceive slowly, remember badly, and seem to be without any but a very feeble impulse to originate ideas for themselves.

Between these two extreme types of children can be found every variety of degree in which the characteristics mentioned above are shown. Children of the first type are usually children with rich natures, endowed with skilful hands and bodies, and good intellects. From these children come the richest and most varied forms of play. Other children who belong to this group, however, are perpetually bothered by the *rush* of ideas and emotions flowing through them, and do not find any form of play satisfying for long. The play of these children, quite apart from any question of emotional stresses and inhibitions, will tend to be shapeless, until such a time as their general age and growth give them vehicles of expression deep enough to hold the composite elements of the thoughts that fill their minds. Earlier in life, ideas occur too frequently, associations are too rich for any form of play to satisfy them for long. This is normal to some forms of childhood, but it can reappear later, when it aproximates to that phenomenon of psychosis known as "flight of ideas".

The second type of child shows exactly opposite characteristics. To such a child ideas come slowly; they carry few associations, and those often poorly and inaccurately formed; he visualises badly and remembers badly, and can move only slowly from idea to idea. The tendency will be for simple pre-existent forms of play to supply adequate expression to such a child. Outlet for his impulses will be better given by forms of play which he can first learn and then repeat, than by those he himself originates. A child of this kind will, therefore, tend to fall fairly readily into existing forms of play, or, having created a form himself successfully once, will feel greater pleasure in repeating this than in attempting to create new games.

This sort of a child feels uncertain in any new situation because his perception of it is poor; and his pleasure in a form of play will often at first be feeble, and gain in strength as he gains in confidence, till the height of pleasure is reached when he feels himself entirely familiar with all aspects of the game and confident in carrying them out. By this time the child of the first type has long exhausted everything that this form of game has to offer him, and feels irritated if he is not allowed to shift to a new game.

Another very powerful factor in the determination of the form of play chosen by children is the relative ease with which a child can detach its interest from a given object and move from object to object.

Human beings vary remarkably in the inborn ease with which their interest or their emotion is able to move from point to point. For reasons which are at present wholly obscure, there appears to be a tendency in certain children to remain fixed in emotional positions once these have been assumed. Such children, once entangled in a situation, find it very difficult to detach their interest or emotion from this position and to move them to other objects or games. They become, as it were, "adherent" to their first choice, and always tend to return to it.

At the other end of the scale, there are children who seem to find a serious difficulty in acquiring a capacity to become sufficiently adherent to any object or experience to enable them properly to assimilate that experience. These children move from object to object with the greatest possible rapidity, and seem to have no capacity for maintaining concentration upon any. It is true that such lack of adhesive qualities may be more apparent than real, and arise from underlying emotional causes, but this fact does not alone account for the type.

This latter type of child may also be the vehicle for a rich flow of ideas, but, though these characteristics do often in fact occur together, it is not necessary for this to be the case. The ideational content of a mind may be poor and yet the fluidity of interest very marked.

When they are extreme, both these types are pathological, but between them, in the region of the normal lies a wide range of difference in the ability either to fix or to shift attention. Children with a tendency to "adhesiveness" fall easily into determined or discreet forms of play; children of the second type spend most of their time in moving from one to another form of play.

The following are examples of both these types:

Children endowed with a rich flow of ideas

E.M., Boy, aged 9. He made a "world" with Indians hunting bison, and a battle between herds of wild animals. There was also a hunt, with fox and hounds. The fox was defended by a tiger, the child remarking that "little things can beat big things." The fox and tiger were then enclosed, and likewise the Indians. There was a battle between Indians, cowboys, and dogs. The dogs turned traitor, half on the side of the Indians and half on the side of the cowboys, and a fight between the pack began.

On another occasion. He staged a fight between two men on a bridge. The one called a "farmer" and the other a "troublesome man". The troublesome man was knocked down, drowned, and buried, and a tombstone was erected: "Here lies a troublesome man." The child remarked, "I know a troublesome girl—my sister. I hate her." The troublesome man then came to life and made love to the farmer's wife. Then there was a second fight, after which a tea-party took place with all actors present, the farmer's wife now nursing a girl child.

On another occasion. Animals were being taken to market, not to be killed, just to change farms, after which the farmer returned home. A motor-cyclist knocked down a Wall's ice-cream man. This was repeated three times. The farmer's wife then stabbed the man in the back. A woman was kidnapped by men and held up for ransom. A forest was then made, and soldiers attacked and penetrated the forest. The trees were thrown down and all the people stood in front to bow. The child said, "It was all a play." The forest was then remade round the two kidnapped women and there was a second battle, E.M. remarking, "It is not a play after all." The women escaped and the police fired into the forest. All the people reappear to bow as before.

On another occasion. A battle of Arabs *v.* Foreign Legion. There was no mass fighting, only duels. The men were then all buried except one, a Foreign Legionary. After this they were all resurrected and the fight resumed, after which there was more burying.

(These four games express very much the same conception set out in several forms.)

L.C., Girl, aged 10. She wrote a story as follows: A tiny crab is caught in an inkwell. It has one friend, a starfish, who is powerless to help it. A small boy tries to get the crab out with two sticks, and drops the inkwell, which smashes. The crab and the starfish then go to the sea. L.C. says first that the crab got into the inkwell when he went to school, and secondly that a lady writing a letter on the sands dropped the inkwell over the crab.

On another occasion. She wrote: three poor orphan boys brought up by a stepfather had often nothing to eat. The father fell ill and was dying, when an old man offered to help them " because they have been good boys to their father." He told them to go into the wood at night and find the biggest and oldest tree, and there they would find something that would save their father's life. The three boys went in different directions, and one found the tree with an owl sitting on it. He called to the other boys to help him move the owl. They found that the owl was sitting on a bag of gold. The boys returned to the village and bought a loaf, and found their father sitting up in bed much better and able to eat the bread. The boys went to the old man and thanked him and gave him part of their gold. They all lived happily ever after.

On another occasion. She made up the following tale: A child in bed wakes up to see three pixies with lights dancing at the foot of her bed. One pixie offers the child three wishes, another pixie says she shall have wishes when she has finished helping her mother wash up next day, and the third pixie says she does not deserve any wishes. The pixies go away and the child is very sad. The next night the first pixie comes and offers the child the wishes again. The child wishes first to live in the country, secondly to go to the pictures, and thirdly that all the family shall live in a big house with a fountain in front, and a swimming-pool. L.C. remarked, " Of course, you couldn't have both the first two wishes, because if you lived in the country you couldn't go to the pictures."

B.G., Boy, aged 5. He began to play with a " world " tray, putting animals two by two in a straight line on a tray without sand, mixing up wild and tame animals together. He had an astonishing knowledge of the animals, and knew them all by name. As he put in the monkey, he said " He is naughty; he is going to jump on to the back of the goat in front of him—he always wants to play tricks." He was most determined to discover all the wild animals that there were in the playroom—searched everywhere, and practically emptied the cabinet containing them, systematically and carefully choosing the ones he wanted. He made a long line of them down the tray to the end, then curved it round the corner of the tray, and, finding a monkey at the head of the line at this point, remarked, " This nasty monkey again! He thinks he is getting food, he is running so, and thinks he is clever. Monkeys always think they are clever, but they are not really. He shall not get anything." He found a dog-kennel and put as many animals inside it as possible. He then put it in the tray so that the animals were marching towards it. When they reached the kennel, worker asked, " Who shall be first?" B.G. said, " Nobody. They are all thinking they will be first." He took a big hedge and put it right in front of the kennel and said, " Nobody is going to come in." He then took the fence away and led the animals past the left side of the kennel, continually asking for more and more wild animals. He said the animals were just having a walk together, and referred frequently to the tiger as "nasty". He added more and more dangerous animals, particularly snakes and crocodiles, and when he had put all these in he said, "No more snakes—they are nasty. All the animals shall die now. You see the snakes poison them." He then told a long story about the snakes who were nasty and were killing all the other animals. He took three people, who, he said, all come from the same home, put them on the edge of the tray, and said it was a zoo and they were watching it. He then took a tank and put two people whom he called father and son at the front and back of it, "and one pulls the gun and aims it, and it makes bang, bang, and all the people are killed." Saying which, he put the tank in the tray, aimed it at the front line of animals and said, "Now they are shooting."

On another occasion. He took square wooden bricks and built what he referred to alternately as a bridge and a tunnel. At first he covered the erection carefully with two bricks and then took them away and tried to expand the bridge at the sides, saying it must be as long as the rails of the train which he had made previously. He called it a "light tunnel" and put odd unsymmetrical triangles on top, and with great concentration played railways with it. At one point in his play he recollected the animal tray with which he had played before and pushed it angrily with his foot, for no apparent reason, so that most of the animals fell down.

On another occasion. He made some long rails for trains with long wooden bricks and found some cars and experimented with them. He continually tried the experiment of putting people in the cars, but decided usually that they were not suitable. He then found an aeroplane and put this on the rails, and experimented with the idea of making it run along them.

On another occasion. Having chosen a tray with sand in it, he took some animals and laid them out in his favourite formation of a queue, two by two—pairs of the same or kindred species being always put together. He then took a tiger, and placed him as last of the queue, with his foreleg on the back of a heavy black hippopotamus, saying, "He is putting his foot right on the hippopotamus, and he'll jump on it in a minute from behind, and the hippopotamus can't run away. it's much too slow and heavy."

Here, on the other hand, are examples of the work of *children with poor ideational endowment.*

G.W., Girl, aged 12½. She asked for a jungle and the sand tray, and made a very civilised jungle, starting with a tin farm and working out the farm idea. At first she was very dependent on worker, asking, "How may cows shall I have?", "How shall I make the jungle, flat or knobbly?", etc. Her imagination of a jungle was very weak, and she spent much time disposing a monkey on a tree, but the monkey kept falling. More attention was given to the monkey than to other beasts. The tray was conventionally divided into a farm and jungle by a straight bank. The jungle was then fenced around, with a passage down the side, and the animals were disposed in a dull pattern everywhere.

On another occasion. She asked to write a story, and wrote as follows:

A WALK

Gertrude: "What have you been doing lately?"
Marguerite: "I have been dancing and enjoying myself."
Gertrude: "Oh, I never have time for that, I have such a lot to do."
Marguerite: "All work and no play makes Jack or anyone a dull boy or girl."
Gertrude: "Oh, don't quote other people—why not be yourself?"
Marguerite: "Well, sometimes it is difficult."
Gertrude: "Let's go bathing."
Marguerite: "Yes, I love diving."
Gertrude: "I don't; it gives me earache."
Marguerite: "I know you like music, but I love dancing—with a really good boy dancer, it's lovely."
Gertrude: "I would just as soon dance alone or with you."
Marguerite: "Heavens, it is time to go home."

A.J., Boy, aged 5. He finds it more difficult each session to decide what he wants to do. To-day he said "No" to hammering and plasticine, when he first arrived, and fell back on water as an old friend because he could not find what else he wanted. He did not play with water for long, and then went in search of the carpentring box. (This was his eighth attendance.)

Here are examples of the child who moves from game to game:

J.J., Boy, aged 8. It was very difficult to get him to settle to anything. Most of the time he wished to wander about and disturb the other children. Water seemed the greatest attraction. He poured several jugs full of water on the sand tray and afterwards he raced boats in the sink.

A.J., Boy, aged 5. He was restless all afternoon, and nothing held his attention for long. He passed from water to Matador, then to plasticine, and back again to water. I tried the zoo, but this did not seem to mean anything to him, except the screws and metal hoofs, which he stuck into long pieces of plasticine. Out of the plasticine he made what he called fish, but these were rolled pieces of different lengths, one very long piece stretching across the table. They had no heads or tails to make them in any way resemble fish.

A.J., Girl, aged 6. She was restless, and changed her occupation often and sometimes with great suddenness. She broke in on other people's occupations, and particularly sought the company of "Doctor".

J.B., Boy, aged 9. He was alert and quick to respond, but restless, and with no apparent wish to carry anything through. He just wandered round looking into everything—cupboards, boxes, etc.

I.S., Girl, aged 9½. She was very restless, continually standing, then sitting, then standing on the seat, and always changing her position. She chewed gum the whole afternoon, doing everything she could think with it— "blowing bubbles", holding it in her teeth, making noises, etc.

These phenomena may verge on the pathological. For example:

M.E., Girl, aged 14. At first she objected to coming with worker. She elected to play draughts after considerable stamping and shouting. She showed a very marked flight of ideas, and incomprehension of the logical or illogical moves, and some spatial confusion. She tended to replace her pieces when they were taken, saying, "Beast! You *are* mean!" Any new stimulus constantly diverted her attention. She quickly tired of draughts.

F.W., Boy, aged 7. He often interrupted his work to gaze round at the others in a vague kind of way. He would not keep his eyes on what he was doing, even when it was a matter of sharpening a pencil (which he did very badly, being too violent and unco-ordinated). During one part of the afternoon he burst suddenly into song.

F.S., Girl, aged 10. She played with the bead mosaics and button mosaics. In each case she merely took all the beads and buttons and arranged them in a solid block with no gaps and no colour arrangement of any kind. She appeared to pick the beads up at random. As soon as she had arranged all the beads, she asked for something else, and refused to try a new pattern. Then she went on to bead threading, which pleased her more than anything else. While working she talked considerably, always seeking to keep my attention when I turned it to someone else. She continually wanted me to admire or praise what she was doing. She was very much interested in, and easily distracted by, what the others were doing. She let her attention wander round the room a great deal, and had continually to be brought back to her own work.

Now, concerning the child who prefers set games or games which he has himself previously devised, some examples of this type will be found in Chapter III in the section devoted to the consideration of ritual, and here are some of the children preferring to play games made up for them by other people:

V.D., Girl, aged 13. She painted outlines on postcards very carefully and well, mixing colours to make the right shades. She did not want to do an original drawing or painting, but asked to copy drawings from the black drawing-book, saying that she did not draw well. These she did with great care and accuracy and quite well.

D.J., Girl, aged 5¾. She showed a certain flatness of manner and dullness of interest. Her mind seemed to run along conventional lines and to express itself in this way if left to itself. Worker stimulated occasionally with suggestions, and drew a creeper growing on the side of a house. D.J. liked it, and said she liked flowers, and added a row of coloured flowers in front of the house. When asked if the house had any chimneys, she said, " Yes ", and drew two.

B.F., Girl, aged 6. When she came in, worker tried to get her to do stencilling, but she insisted on doing a picture puzzle which she knew. She did it with boasts—" You thought I couldn't do it." She was careless, and did not put the pieces in accurately, then said, " I can't do this. You do it." Later she insisted on being read to from a book that she knew, and refused all creative work.

A third factor in the determination of the shape of play is the question of the *suitability of the material available.* It would appear at first sight that restlessness and dissatisfaction displayed in a child when surrounded by a roomful of toys *must* arise from some defect or fault in the child itself. But careful study of this problem has convinced the writer that, while this is sometimes true, it is by no means invariably the case. The same result may be produced by the opposite causes.

Children who desire to achieve a certain sort of expression, and are profoundly absorbed by a certain sort of problem, if they cannot find material suitable for the expression of that idea, or the working out of that problem, may be unable to play at all until they can. Thus a child surrounded by Meccano, toy trains, dolls, picture-books, and jig-saws, who has in his mind a dominant problem concerning the nature of earth and water, will moon about among the toys, trying first one and then another, and discarding each in turn because of the absence of water and earth. Thus shapelessness and restlessness in play may be due not to the indefiniteness, but to the very *definiteness* of the form of the idea in a child's mind. In this case it arises from the child's inability to find material which fits both its power of expression and the form of the idea to be expressed. A child in this state is in the same position as a versatile artist with a half-formed conception in his mind, who finds himself without the proper medium for he expression of his idea. For example, if the following child had been in a playroom unfurnished with water it is difficult to see what she would have done, and water is rarely available for play in a nursery.

G.S., *Girl, aged 7¾.* She was busy cleaning the dolls' house when I came to her. This she continued industriously, washing the windows again and again, and placing the furniture neatly in the rooms. Although she is Jewish, she said she was getting the house ready for Christmas. In the dining-room three people sat at table. G.S. said she had many dolls at home, one named Ted, a teddy-bear named Pat, a china doll named Manie, three Dutch dolls, Stella, Kitty, and Tommy, and two or three more. Presently the whole house was very thoroughly washed. Then, noticing a group next door, playing house on the floor with much elaborate equipment, she became interested in them. At first she threw water at one of the girls, then after a bit asked if she might play with their things. They assented, and she took flour and water, secured sand for cocoa and proceeded to make it. Going to the sink for water, she became interested in playing there with another girl, using water running through a funnel inserted into the end of the hose. She played with this till the time to go home., She was industrious, uncommunicative, less talkative than usual, and quiet except for the one incident of sprinkling water on another girl, and used water throughout the afternoon and for every aspect of her play.

Some children even definitely refuse material which is offered to them, and yet do not know what they want. For instance:

G.W., *Girl, aged 12.* (A new girl.) She was rather shy and diffident, and a little supercilious. She was not interested in our material, asked if that was all, and wasn't she going to have a treatment. She put mosaic pieces tentatively together, but said she could not do it and jumbled them up.

M.E., *Girl, aged 12.* She opened several boxes to see what there was and said she was too old for bricks, and could not do mosaics or Meccano. She asked for plasticine, but when she got it she did not know what to do with it.

P.T., *Boy, aged 4.* He refused to make a "world", and appeared not to understand what to do with it. He took handfuls of animals and buried them indiscriminately. He picked out a snake, which alone seemed to attract him, and asked questions about it. Then he put it on the elephant's trunk, and finally flung it across the room. Worker put houses into the sand, but they did not interest him.

Even if all possible forms of material be present, the problem is not necessarily solved, Many children need to make many false attempts in different forms of material before they find the one that is suitable to express their ideas. To the outside observer, an afternoon spent in this way often appears to have passed in aimless muddle, but under the surface it has had its purpose, and has been expressive of definite thought and direction. All these points are worthy of being borne in mind in evaluating "shapeless play ".

We now come back to our first point; what makes a child play by himself or with his fellows? It is not sufficient to say of a child that he " refuses to play in a group ", for some children will play with a group when a particular rôle is alloted to them, but will not otherwise play at all. Some children will only play if certain rôles are *not* allotted to them and, for example, shrink to the wall if asked to take the lead. An illustration of this has been given in G.D.'s report on page 172. Here are some more:

K.T., Boy, aged 7. His reaction to the " enemy " when the " house " was being attacked was to hide behind chairs when they were arriving. He made no attempt to resist or attack the enemy, and took no initiative in leading the others or guarding them or the house. When all the others had made their escape, he also escaped and ran out to the rocking-horse, on which he said he was riding away.

D.S., Girl, aged 11. She tended to keep in the background and leave the lead to others. Before the game began she had been hiding with a boy and a girl behind the curtains at the back of the piano. She did not want to join in the game of statues, but afterwards she was reluctantly persuaded to do so.

Some children, on the contrary, will act or take part in group games only if they are given the leading rôle. For example:

K.T., Boy, aged 7. While playing charades with three older girls, he was a bit at a loose end at first, and not quite in his element. When asked to take the lead and be a captain of a boat, he was overjoyed, and entered into the whole thing heart and soul. He did not boss things too much, but just felt he was someone for the time being. He played very well in the group.

I.S., Girl, aged 9½. When playing charades she showed herself to be the born leader. She organised the charade and managed the other children, although she was the youngest present.

B.C., Girl, aged 10½. When playing with the dolls' house with L.C. (Girl, aged 10), she at once assumed the rôle of leader, organising and arranging everything, and expecting worker to wait on her. They played as follows: Two mothers lived together, with their husbands at work and with children to look after. They cleaned out the rooms and washed the floors, which extended to washing and polishing the floor of the playroom and the table. Dinner was then prepared, served, and eaten, and cakes were made. During the whole time B.C. always took the lead, and at first resented L.C.'s showing any originality. For example, when L.C.'s baby was two months old, B.C.'s was at once one month old. When L.C. made a special kind of tart, B.C. declared she had thought of it too. Worker pointed out that all the cakes were different, and all equally interesting and good. B.C. finally was quite pleased by this, but scored by getting some extra dough, which she stole from a boy, and made three cakes to L.C.'s two.

G.W., Girl, aged 13. G.W. and L.C. were doing charades. G.W. was eager to participate when her word was being performed and showed considerable aptitude in making up conversations into which the word or syllable was brought. When it came to L.C.'s turn, G.W. complained that her head hurt and was altogether thoroughly unco-operative.

M.E., Girl, aged 14. M.E. and F.V. (Girl, aged 7) were acting a play of Princess, Rajah, and disguised Prince. M.E. as Rajah was directing and bossing heavily. Worker as Princess was told what to do and discouraged from playing the part too freely. When M.E. went out, the others were told to sit and talk till she came back. But as she was a long time, worker encouraged F.V. to run away with her. When M.E. came back there was a mix-up of Rajah and Prince riding on horses, shooting, hands up, and then Rajah and Prince were confederates, and M.E. called F.V. to hurry worker away to execution by hanging.

Some children will play only if a particular other child is present. For instance:

M.C., Girl, aged 13. At the sight of M.R., a girl aged 11, she wanted to join her, and remained seated on the floor playing house with her for the rest of the afternoon, apart from a rather reluctant visit to Mrs. X. (dancing). The only thing that roused her was the suggestion that she should leave M.R., and then she definitely refused to move.

On another occasion. On the way to the playroom she asked if M.R. was there, and repeated this at intervals till M.R. came. Then she rushed over to her and asked if she was going to dress up. M.R. shook her head, and M.C. returned to the table and did not refer to M.R. or to dressing up again.

M.E., Girl, aged 14. She constantly asked after G., and, on being told that she was busy, accepted the deprivation of her society quite well, She asked repeatedly if she might go with G. to the rhythm room, but again accepted quite docilely the statement that everybody had to have their own turn, and that she could go at the end, but was without interest for the whole of the afternoon.

B.C., Girl, aged 10½. She began to show anxiety as to whether L.C. would come, and expressed an urgent need for a companion in play. Worker asked if this was "because L.C. does what you tell her to?" B.C.: "No because it's nice to have someone to play with." There were several other girls in the room.

G.W., Girl, aged 12¾. She asked if she could play skittles with B.C., and told worker later on that this was what she had planned to do this afternoon. She wanted to know if this arrangement could always hold, but was told if could not, since she and B.C. had things to do alone sometimes. She did not accept B.C.'s suggestion of naming the skittles, nor appear to mind being beaten. She was always ready to find balls and put the skittles in order. She wanted to go on with this game until she saw that B.C. wished a change.

Some children, as is well known, play better in the presence of one adult, and remain shy and inhibited if their friend be absent. Here are some examples:

J.D., Girl, aged 5. She noticed some of the other children dressing up, and asked if she could join. Some clothes were found, and she chose a green and white costume which worker called "Maid Marion". Three others were in costumes, and they were asked to act. J.D. became very frightened, and could hardly answer worker. She almost wanted to hide behind her to keep out of the way. Miss X. then joined in, and they were dressed up by the children, J.D. choosing the most gorgeous robe she could find for worker. When Miss X. was there J.D. joined in well with a birthday party and dance game.

M.J., Girl, aged 7. She was happily excited, and entered into the game both as actor and watcher in the charades, but she did not want to initiate anything by herself. Mrs. Z. and worker did it, too, and she joined in quite happily. She followed I.S.'s lead while playing statues, and did not want to do things alone. When worker was with her, she joined in happily.

M.R., Girl, aged 11. As worker approached her in the parents' room, she stiffened, looked terrified, then flushed and hung her head. Worker ignored this, and in about fifteen seconds M.R. took her hand and came into the playroom quite calmly. On the stairs M.R. again got her "fixed" expression, flushed painfully, and worker, thinking she was going to cry, suggested that she would be sorry to hear of the absence of Mrs. Z. with whom she had played before. After this M.R. was soon chatting naturally. She asked if she might continue last Friday's game with P.S. She asked worker not to leave her for more than a minute.

Some children will play only in a group large enough to lose themselves in, and some, frightened by a large group, will play well only with a small set of children.

Some will play running games and refuse to join in quiet ones. For example:

G.W., Girl, aged 13. (Referred for backwardness and lack of concentration.) She wanted to play ball, but this was impossible to-day. She then refused to play anything else, and said she was too old for the games here, though she had enjoyed them when she first came. She did not want to sit in the playroom, so we sat on the stairs. Conversation was very desultory, and she was very bored. Once she said, "Oh, do let's do something interesting", but had no suggestions and did not like any of worker's suggestions.

On another occasion. She was undecided what to do, and accepted drawing and began a Christmas card without much enthusiasm. She said she did not like sitting still, and would like to do things that kept her moving all the time. She spoke with interest of the games they played in school, particularly rounders, and remarked that it was no fun doing things alone.

Some children, on the other hand, will join a group for a quiet game, and become moody and solitary when asked to run about.

Others will enjoy a game with a thrill in it (e.g. "Steps" or "Blind Man's Buff"), while some are made miserable by this sort of suspense.

Many children will play uproariously games of their own choice, and become sulky when asked to join in games made up by someone else. For instance:

G.W., Girl, aged 9. She took no interest at all in the play we did on a theme suggested by R.F. She only wanted to play at school. As soon as we started this she became intensely domineering and almost bullying in her manner, but when A.J. and R.F. did pictures at her command, it was interesting to note that the artist in her was stronger than the autocrat. "Those are very good", she said, quite enthusiastically. However, when R.F. meekly asked if she might have good marks, the reply was immediate and firm: "Infants don't have marks."

G.W., Girl, aged 13. She restricted herself to physical exercise, high kicking against my hand, which exhilarated her very much, and "walking down the wall" by bending over backwards till her palms touched the wall and then seeing how far down it she could pass her hands, etc. She was unwilling to settle to any other occupation.

Some children like to turn everything into acting.

I.S., Girl, aged 9. She is a very good little actress, and thoroughly enjoys it. She recited some poetry and was quite in her element. She was *the* person, and appreciated it. She was happy when acting with the others, and made her story for acting well as she went along. Nothing else interested her as much.

J.P., Girl, aged 8½. This child insisted upon acting in season and out of season. She required no encouragement to act for her plans were absolutely clear in her mind. She explained to worker that her play needed four people; a Prince, a Princess, a King, and a Queen. She would play the rôle of Prince. The Prince and Princess were quarrelling about a baby doll, and both tugged at it to try to get hold of it. Finally they made up the quarrel, and the Prince sang a love song and the " Kiss Waltz " to the Princess. A banquet and a party followed. The banquet was followed by a variety entertainment to which each contributed. J.P. was very quick to see possibilities for utilising nursery rhymes she had sung and dramatised with worker earlier. The final scene was a wedding, with appropriate music.

On another occasion. She started to dress up with bits of stuff, putting a piece of net across her forehead and eyes. Later she discarded this and had only a piece of stuff across her forehead. She called herself a Princess, and dressed her doll as a Princess also. She went downstairs to act with two other girls. At first the others organised the proceedings, but J.P. acted her parts well and insisted that the King should recognise her as his daughter and not treat her as a stranger, as he was inclined to do.

On another occasion. While acting *Cinderella*, she took the part of the Prince, acting it well. Acting appeals to this child; she quickly becomes identified with the part, and has a certain imaginative capacity for carrying it out. She gets excited and anxious for the play as a whole, telling the others what to do, and showing a wish to stage-manage and organise, but is not really capable of dealing with the situation.

Certain children, on the contrary, refuse to act at all.

E.R., Boy, aged 11. He got out a Chinese coat and showed it to worker, but did not put it on. He referred to dressing-up as " a girl's game ", and made disparaging references to girls.

M.B., Girl, aged 9. She found a group dressing up, but refused to join in. She sat in a corner on the pram, watching the others. Every time they urged her to join them, she refused abruptly. Finally she did become interested in the garments, but did not attempt to dress up, merely looked at the things. She picked up a feather fan, handled it, stroked worker's face with it, then used it as a duster and finally threw it back on the heap of garments.

Some will act only if there is an audience.

G.W., Girl, aged 14. She asked at once for the dressing-up box. Worker was Father Christmas, and she was his wife. She did not appear to have any conception of a set story, saying, " You must make it up as you go along." Her part was full of grandiose artificial phrases and expressions, her gestures occasionally reminiscent of the stage and very exaggerated. *She demanded an audience,* and would not be in without one. The play consisted of: (*a*) preparations for Father Christmas's journey, which was to Scotland, and (*b*) the return home, Christmas being over.

J.B., Boy, aged 6. He put on the brightest clothes he could find, long stockings and a lady's riding-hat. He opened a sunshade and strutted about, telling worker to go and fetch someone to come and look at him, which happened to be impossible and undesirable. J.B. then sat on the floor for some time, quietly playing with the sunshade, then he got out the long black skirt, which he made into a sort of tent, getting right inside it so that he was completely hidden. He again said, " Go and get someone to come and look at me ", but when he found worker did not do so, he took off the clothes and put them away.

But an audience does not appeal to everyone, as this little girl shows:

D.C., Girl, aged 4. The door was open and the gramophone was audible from the rhythm room. In Dr. L.'s room D.C. felt herself alone, and began to dance away to herself very gracefully and in time to the music. At first she did not see me, but as soon as she did she stopped dancing, and we have never been able to get her to dance since.

Now, it should be noted that these differences in behaviour are not accidental.

In a paper by Charlotte Bühler[51], evidence is brought together to substantiate a suggestion that there are essential and primary differences in the general disposition of children to society. Dr. Bühler suggests that there are three normal types of social behaviour in children: the socially blind infant, the socially dependent infant, and the socially independent infant. The difference between them is brought out by their behaviour in the presence of another child. In such a situation the first type of child behaves as if no one were present. " He does not pay any attention to the other's movements; he is neither impressed nor interested " in the activity of other children.

The socially dependent child, on the contrary, is deeply affected by the presence of other children. He may be inhibited or stimulated, but, whichever be the effect, all his movements are dependent upon the movements of other children. Throughout his contact with another child, he observes the effect of his behaviour upon the other child, and the other child's reactions to him.

The socially independent child is the child who is aware of the presence of other children and responsive to them, but neither dependent, intimidated, nor inspired. He may or may not join the other in play, but, whichever it may be, he remains independent, and his co-operation depends always upon initiative from within himself, and not upon the effect upon him of the other children's thoughts or actions.

"These three types", says Charlotte Bühler, "were observed with infants from six to about eighteen months of age. They occurred independently of whether or not the children had had previous contacts with others, also independently of whether or not they were only children, independently also of their home conditions, and even of their nationalities. . . Some of these babies were retested in several contacts with older and younger, superior and inferior, children, and seemed not to vary in their typical disposition and attitude."

It would therefore seem from this evidence that these attitudes are primary dispositions, and are not dependent upon environment.

As concerns the relationship of individuals in groups to the group, Dr. Bühler distinguished also four types:

1. *The Leader.* Many studies have been made by several observers establishing the fact of essential leadership in certain children, and analyses have been made of the nature of the qualities that make for leadership.[52,53] Several examples already quoted demonstrate this kind of child.

2. *The Popular Child.* This is a child who is not necessarily a leader at all, and very often has many of the opposite characteristics to those of leadership, but he contains in himself qualities which are spontaneously attractive to his fellows. "All children seem to like him; they wish to sit near him and to serve him." Every group of children contains one or more of this kind of child. Clearly such a child would not find his way to the Institute.

3. *The Protective Type.* A child of this sort seeks always another child to whom he can become protective. When one child ceases to need his protection and passes out of that situation, the protective child will always look for another to whom he can extend aid. He is only really at peace when he is actively caring for someone else. For example:

D.J., Girl, aged 9¾. She was very yielding with the little ones, and put her arm round a younger child maternally.

D.D., Girl, aged 10. B.H. joined the game, and was unhappy and on the verge of tears. D.D. immediately started mothering her, and put her arm round her and tried to coax her to do things with her. Later on she was a little shocked when B.H. said she did not want to do something, and said, "Oh, Beth!" reproachfully.

4. *The socially unsuccessful child.* "The neglected and poor child, whose dress is torn and dirty, or the child with physical defects, is socially unsuccessful, as well as always the mischief-maker, the quarrelsome child, and the one who always knows better."[51] For example:

F.V., Girl, aged 7. She was rude and difficult and mischievous all the afternoon, specially towards the children, pulling their hair, smacking and pinching them. She took a difficult jig-saw, and quite welcomed worker at first, but when worker interfered with her smacking the other children, F.V. became noisy and rude and made faces.

But there should also be added to this group of types that of the essential follower, the Boswell of children. Every group of children tends to contain a certain number who form the lieutenants, or the essential "members" of the group. Such children are never leaders, never particularly popular, rarely protective, and never unsuccessful socially. They form the main bulk of many groups, and are essentially children most happy in the company of leaders, and when forming one of a group whose spirit they catch and whose actions they copy. Here are some examples from the Institute:

J.D., Girl, aged 5. She refused to go to dancing and slid under the table. B.F. was eager to dance, and at her invitation J.D. went too. Once outside the playroom, the situation altered, J.D. pulling B.F. along. On the previous occasion J.D. had refused to dance, but had gone willingly at the invitation of the other children.

On another occasion. She went to the water room because it was familiar, but had no definite idea of application, and said deliberately to I.S., "I am going to copy you." I.S. proceeded with her baby-washing phantasy, and J.D. deliberately copied everything she did.

M.R., Girl, aged 11. She was rather subdued and shy, and watched another girl's assertive behaviour as if rather alarmed by it. She played second fiddle to another girl quite contentedly all afternoon.

There is also the child whose relation to the group is always that of jester or buffoon (see Chapter IX). The following examples describe typical behaviour of certain children:

M.R., Girl, aged 11. She played house game, and until closing time seemed

quite calm and happy and did not show any excitement, but then she and
M.C. (a girl) turned their faint attempts at clearing up into a " rag ". They
rushed about the room and passages, dabbling everyone with wet and
doughy hands, and thoroughly enjoying the good-humoured reaction of
the adults.

G.S., Girl, aged 7¾, and M.J., Girl, aged 7. They were mixing a porridge-like
mess to which plasticine currants were added. G.S. pretended to taste it,
then put the spoon in worker's mouth with such suddenness that worker
perforce ate some. This caused great merriment to both children, and
G.S. began smacking worker's face with her doughy hands, and shook bits
off them towards M.J.

These attitudes to society, once formed, tend to be stable, and the child
can co-operate with a group at play only so long as he is allowed to occupy
his given natural rôle in relation to the group. Sections A and D of Chapter
II, and Susan Isaacs' study of the *Social Development in Young Children*[31] give
many examples of this kind of temperament. Children of the types
described by Dr. Bühler early codify their relationship to the outside world,
and will only co-operate with it when they can force it to fall within their own
pattern of behaviour. Such children appear to bring to life a pre-arranged
pattern of behaviour, and are only able to take part in life when it falls into
this predetermined shape.

The underlying rule of all these types of reaction to play is that *the form of
play chosen must represent to the child the phantasies he is at the moment conceiving,
or must give vent to the bodily desires by which he feels himself moved.*

This brings us to our last point: how does it come about that some
children, healthy in body and of normal intellect, fail absolutely to play at
all? If play in children were an instinct, as is play in kittens, such cases should
not occur.

Children showing inhibitions in all forms of play fall into four classes:

1. The children who have been considered already and who will play
games only on their own terms.

2. Children who are unable or unwilling to play any specific form of
play, but who nevertheless will indulge in spontaneous play of their own
devising.

3. Children who are unable to initiate or join in *any* form of play
whatever.

4. Shy children, who cannot join in or initiate any games while with
strangers, but who join in well as soon as they become accustomed to their
surroundings.

It is regrettable that the reading which has been done for this book has brought to light no study of the incidence of these forms of inhibition in play among any group of children, and we can therefore only consider the groups upon general principles.

Class 1 we have already considered. Let us take as an illustration of *Class 2* a girl of four years old, a third child of three children, of intelligent parents and a cultured home. She was brought for treatment owing to her inability to mix with her fellows in a nursery school. While the other children took part in the ordinary life of the school, Winnie would sit apart in a corner, playing with her hands.

Winnie's play with her hands was first described by her mother, who said that Winnie would pretend her hands were flies, one doing things that the other did not approve of, and being punished. Sometimes one " fly " would get squashed by the other and be bandaged or taken to hospital, and mother's hands were occasionally called in to play the rôle of doctor, of a " nice man helping poor ' Little Fly ' " and so on.

She played the game several times at the Institute in conjunction with toys. On the first occasion, while she was painting, Winnie suddenly began to make one hand run up and down the table, saying that it was " Little Fly " who had got his legs burnt, "though there was no fire." This may have referred to her own legs, as she reported that she had burnt herself that morning. Once, while playing at lavatories with her dolls, she made " Little Fly " defæcate, and on another occasion he was made to drive a car and run over a paper ball. " Little Fly " sometimes occupied her attention for longer periods, being cradled like a doll, washed meticulously, and given tea. Another time, worker had some difficulty in making her wash her hands before leaving, because this would mean a bath for " Little Flies ".

Here the crucial obstacle blocking this child's capacity to join in play with companions was the dominant nature of her own phantasy. This held her attention to such a degree that it left no interest free to be devoted to other pursuits. As in the case considered above, the child is obsessed with problems that play themselves out continually in her head, and for the expression of which other children are not a suitable medium.

There are many cases of this kind. The boy in Chapter V, pages 112–113, was a boy who had shown himself to be unable to combine with boys in any way, and who was terrified of meeting boys in a group. Yet, when alone with one worker, this boy showed very abundant ideas, good power of representation, and patience in working out his conceptions. His own emotional problems were too dominant to allow him sufficient freedom of mind to wish to join in the games of other children.

Class 3 is in its causes a special example of this general rule. The children of this group form an absorbingly interesting study. Many of them are children who are inhibited from any form of play at all. An example of the degree to which this refusal can be carried is given in the following extracts:

D.C., Girl, aged 4. She arrived with her mother and progressed as far as the office door, and began to cry. She was carried downstairs to a room off the playroom by a worker, and for the next hour and twenty minutes she cried continually, at intervals stamping her feet in fury. All the ordinary things in which she had shown any interest so far were put ready for her, within easy reach, but she refused to take the smallest notice of them, hiding herself as far as possible in the corner of the room, with her face to the wall. At intervals the cries began to subside, but they were always renewed at any attempt to make contact with her, or to get her interested in any activity. There was definite advance to-day in that once or twice she hit out with annoyance at certain things offered to her, actually recognising their presence. Hitherto she has entirely refused to externalise her annoyance in any way. After about an hour and a half her cries began to shape themselves into words, and became resolved into a demand for her mother to come downstairs. This was met, as similar demands had been in previous sessions, by an assurance that her mother was quite well and happy, was upstairs, was busy reading, and that she could go to her as soon as the afternoon was over, or could go and see her at any moment if she cheered up and stopped crying. At the end of the afternoon she wandered about the downstairs corridor, hanging about the open door of the playroom, obviously wanting to go in, but not being able to allow herself to venture.

On another occasion. She arrived with her mother and burst into tears as she got into the library. She neither refused nor agreed to come downstairs and, partly carrying and partly gently urging her, she was induced to come downstairs, howling loudly all the while. She spent the whole time in my room, yelling hard for half the afternoon, then she stopped and stood about the room, but did not use the toys at all.

K.W., Boy, aged 11. (Referred to the Institute for stammering.) (First visit.) A very sweet shy child. He sat at a table against the wall and facing it. On his right was the cabinet of animals, and he kept his back to worker, who was on his left, while choosing animals from the cabinet, only turning slightly towards the tray when placing the objects, which he did without any plan. He gave a shut-away impression: his movements were indrawn and careful, neat and precise. He carefully shook the sand away from an object before putting it down, and he always put things away as he finished with them. Every question I put to him brought him round towards me a little, until he gained confidence to be openly eager about and pleased with what he did, and towards the end he laughed openly when pleased. At first he had given only the ghost of a smile.

R.A., Girl, aged 3. She left her mother, and sucked her thumb vigorously, totally absorbed in this activity. She paid little attention to coloured bricks offered to her. Worker drew her hands down gently and she did not resist, but went on sucking her lips with intense absorption in this sensation to the point of trembling. She ran her hands over her lips as if sucking an orange, and stood thus, refusing to pay attention to any of the play materials available.

M.M., Boy, aged 2. He was entirely negative and resentful and finally cried uproariously for his mother. As all attempts to distract him seemed to accentuate his annoyance, worker appeared to ignore him and played with water and a plasticine figure. After a while M.M. stopped screaming and took a very half-hearted interest in what was going on. He noticed other children playing in the garden, but showed no inclination to join them. After standing with his hands behind his back, like a thoroughly disgruntled man, he peevishly asked worker to move a jar of water, and then to empty part of its contents, then, becoming calmer, he accepted the proposal to explore the water room.

The subsequent development of these children while under treatment at the Institute proves that these failures to combine with other children, or to develop spontaneous play, do not arise from any inherent absence in the child of the capacity for play, or to any lack of interior power to externalise ideas.

D.C., on a later occasion. She came into the garden and began playing with skittles, knocking them down, kicking the box, and hurling them finally at the wall. One skittle she mischievously threw over the wall, but agreed that it was better not to throw any others. She then came indoors to the shop and played for some time with paper bags and flour. She seemed to enjoy this very much, and later went to the water room. There she dabbled about with a mop, and then began chasing worker and running after her full pelt, regardless of other people's presence. She wet part of the water room, remarking, " I am making all this wet, so you can't get over it." Every time worker came near D.C., she chased her, ran into the garden, covered the mop with mud and ran back, chasing worker all round with it.

On another occasion. She was in the water-room and invented a game which consisted of making soap-suds in the sink, and then hiding the scrubbing-brush, soap, or rag under the suds and asking worker where it was. Worker and D.C. made a careful search, and pretended to be very surprised when the hidden objects were discovered. When she found that worker's suds had gone cold, she became quite concerned, and generously gave some from her own bowl. She called the suds "snow", and seemed immensely to enjoy the experience of playing with them.

K.W., on a later occasion. He asked at once for a model aeroplane made last time. It was to have a trial flight to-day; the pilot would take up two passengers. He was in the Air Force, and also piloted for Imperial Airways. The two important people sat in front, the friend at the back with the luggage, and the flight was to be to Lympne. Everything was successful and the pilot was much praised by the passengers.

R.A., on a later occasion. She was playing with moist sand, patting it. She then made a house with a chimney by piling up an empty match-box and a tin pot. She made mounds of sand, and poked holes in it with a clay stick and her fingers. She asked for water and the toy lavatory, and filled it continually. Then she dropped some "dirt" (as she called clean sand) into it. She filled the watering-can and watered the garden. She filled an empty teacup with water from the teapot, and made a cup of tea which she emptied into the lavatory. She played with water for about ten minutes. She took the things out of the box and arranged them on the table, naming them as she found them. She called the kangaroo a rabbit, and when she found the rabbit, which rather resembled the kangaroo, she asked where the baby was. When she had looked at all the animals she helped to put them away. She was given drawers containing people, transport, trees, grass, and a dry sand tray, and she proceeded to make a hill and asked, "What goes on a hill?" She heaped the sand into a high mound and dotted trees over it, put fences at the base, and grouped all the transport together in "the road". She had quite a good idea of arrangement. Finding in a corner "grass" for the cow and sheep, she put all the pigs together, the mother pig with the baby pigs. She seated two figures on a stile. A curious feature of her play was the repeated act of burying something. For example, a goose was poked into the sand, and later fetched out again.

On another occasion. She made a garden with trees, and wanted flowers, saying she loved flowers. She watered them all with a watering-can and water. Then she found three ladders and put them by the side of the sand tray, and then put men on the top to look over the garden wall. Next she found a teapot and wanted to put water in it.

M.M. on a later occasion. There was some sand in the big boat and he got some on his hands. He washed this off very carefully and asked for his hands to be dried. He touched the back of a large red duck and said, "Pink", then he touched another duck and said, "Pink". He wanted to float the large duck, and was irritated because there was no room. He then asked for the toy pump, but, as he could not work it well, he was not very much interested in it. Then he asked for the " wee-wee place ". He tried to lift the seat, but as it was stiff he could not do so. He was irritated, and asked worker to do it. He made the things work, putting his finger down the bowl, and said, " Wee-wee down there ", and " Ugh-ugh down there." He pointed to the wash-basin he wanted, first one and then the other (there were only two). He wanted these filled continually, and showed worker which tap to turn, generally wanting first one and then the other.

It is clear, therefore, that the failures to play shown at the beginning of treatment do not lie in any lack of interest in play, or capacity to originate ideas.

The cause of this failure lies elsewhere. Most children, we have seen, have a very active phantasy life, but it is of a kind that is very difficult to express in words. Moreover, many of their ideas and imaginations are concerned with a mixture of experience and concept which are unacceptable to the world around them, and particularly is this true of ideas of aggression and destruction.

Some of the hostilities they feel, as we have seen in Chapter IV, lie near the surface, and are expressible without too much difficulty by fairly direct symbolic play. Some, however, lie far deeper, and are totally inaccessible to any direct form of expression. Too little work has been done upon this problem for any exhaustive knowledge of the causes of these conditions to be available, but some suggestions can be put forward. In some cases it appears that hostile emotions exist which are felt by the individual to be so dangerous in quality that no form of expression is possible or permissible. A parallel to this situation in children is the phrase heard from time to time on the lips of adults—" I was so afraid of what I might say, that I said nothing at all." It is often possible in the play of children during their early days at the Institute actually to see this connection between inhibition and hostility. For example:

J.D., Girl, aged 5. Repeatedly this afternoon J.D. said to suggested activities, " I don't want to ", and lost interest to the point of seeming futility, when an activity, which she expected not to be allowed to do, was allowed. Several times when passing a table she stretched out her hand and deliberately destroyed something someone had made or was making.

G.S., Girl, aged 7¾. She would not settle down with anything for the first half-hour or so. She first flitted about from one thing to another, blew soap-bubbles, then wandered about and went over to the sand, just turned that over, then went to the water tray and filled two jugs, one of which she poured over her own sand and then over another child's work. She then ran across the room and destroyed the "world" another child was making.

Hostility in children can take such an extreme form, and be associated with a child's other emotions in such a way as to be utterly terrifying to the child himself, and provision of suitable material for expression will then be regarded by the child as a threat rather than as an offer of help. Such children can only acquiesce in the destructive acts of other people.

If such aggressive permissions be wisely and impersonally given, and the whole child is encircled at the same time with an atmosphere of safety, it can be led step by step out of its self-created prison of hostility and its natural impulse to play set free, as for example with the following child:

J.D., Girl, aged 5. She came in with her finger in her mouth. She was given a "world", as she had liked it the previous time. She put a few animals out without any apparent purpose and was very bored. She asked to paint. She always appears to want something that someone else has got, and to try to take it from the possessor. Later she began a picture puzzle, and was quite animated at first, but became bored as soon as she was alone. When I joined her she cheered up, and picked up a roll of paper and started tapping people. First she did this gently, then harder, becoming violently aggressive. After doing this a while, Dr. L. told me to give her baby doll to hit, and at once there was a real transformation. She nursed the baby with every appearance of love, holding it beautifully. She looked at another doll in the box, and with a knowing look pointed out the bare bottom of a small doll. Then she asked for the bed, made it carefully, and put the doll in it. When it was time to go, she helped me to fold up the bed and put it away. This was very different from her usual spiteful behaviour.

M.M., Boy, aged 2. He had been playing quite nicely with his sister, and when she left him he started to follow her. Worker then sat on the stairs in front of him and tried to distract his attention, whereupon he began to howl, and this soon changed to a bellow. He howled loudly, crying, "Mummy! Mummy! Upstairs! Gar-gar upstairs!" and pointing to himself and saying, "Upstairs." Worker began building up some large bricks on the stairs, and after a minute he began to knock them down. He knocked down several, and then refused to do so any more. Another child came along, and M.M. struck out at him. He clung on to worker, hoping she would take him to his mother. Dr. L. came and sat on the stairs too, and made a plasticine "mummy", and with the worker began to pull it to bits. M.M. continued to cry, but became quite interested. Dr. L. asked him if we should pull off the middle or the head. He stopped crying long enough to say, "Head", and went on whimpering. When the plasticine was all pulled to bits, worker sat on the floor by the door and made another "mummy", which was pulled to bits. By M.M.'s orders the skirt was taken off first. Then worker and M.M. made his sister and pulled her to bits. M.M. then took a lump of yellow plasticine and picked up a man with a gun and began to dig the gun into the plasticine, saying, "Daddy." Then he went to another child and put the gun in her mouth. There were no more tears this afternoon.

Hostility can also be expressed symbolically.

R.A., Girl, aged 3. She began playing with rabbits, and buried them one by one—father, mother, and little girl and baby rabbit—and, when asked why, she said because they had spilt something over the tortoise. She then became wildly excited and destructive, and these two moods alternated. She buried figures symbolising other people, and seemed to be possessed with a kind of demoniac energy to destroy the work of other children.*

Careful and persistent following-up of aggressive themes results in steady loosening of the inhibition to play and a frank expression of aggression in action. For example:

R.A., on another occasion. I went to fetch water for her, and she knocked down everyone else's things. When I had to write and could not play with her, she knocked me and said I was naughty, and she went on being as destructive as possible towards other people's things. She then went "mad dog" through the Institute. She knocked down her own blocks and also those of a boy, which amused him, and then the two played at throwing things about. The was a great deal of noise, R.A. being the ringleader. (R.A. later developed into a charming and friendly little girl with an excellent play sense.)

We come now to the last variety of inhibitions in children.

Class 4. Children who are too shy to play. This kind of inability to play in a group may be due to:

(*a*) Lack of proper start in life and lack of experience of other children.
(*b*) Unusual poverty of ideas or slowness of mind.
(*c*) The phenomenon we call shyness.

(*a*) *Lack of a proper start in life.* Sociability, as is the case with all other qualities, needs experience. The child who has been for the greater part of his life alone is without experience of contact with other human beings. He does not know *how* to play, and has to be taught. Every nursery-school teacher who draws her pupils from among isolated only children will have had experience of this phenomenon.

---

*It is interesting to note that about this time her headmistress wrote: " It was with great pleasure that I noted the change for the better in R.A. A few weeks ago she refused to help in the social work—to-day willingly agreed to help. She sensibly packed all the milk money ready for the milkman, and went with another girl to every classroom with the numbers for the week. She was laughing, happy, and kind all the time."

(*b*) *The slow child.* Children who grasp a new idea with great difficulty often find it practically impossible to play with a group with which they are unfamiliar. The speed of thought of the other children, and the type of ideas they express, make demands on his mental capacity that he cannot satisfy. Only when he is thoroughly familiar with both the game and the group with which he is playing is he really able to play his part adequately.

(*c*) *Shyness.* Shyness is a very curious phenomenon, and closely associated with ego-centricity. The shy child is either a timid child, a child who shrinks from contact with strangers owing to a real fear of his fellows, or a child with a phantasy picture of himself which is deeply precious to him and to which he fears the others will not do justice. Shy children, like shy adults, usually have unconsciously a very high opinion of their value, and hesitate to join a group or move out of their isolation, lest the touchstone of reality prove their dream to be but phantasy.

The following are examples from the I.C.P. playroom reports of shy children:

P.T., Boy, aged 4. Worker went with him to dancing. He watched other boy with interest, but kept his eye on the open door by which he could escape to familiar surroundings. Twice, when urged to join in, he ran to the door and whimpered, "Mummy", but interest drew him back and at last he volunteered to run with the others. Greatly daring, he ran through the further room into the yard and paddled in a puddle.

A.U., Boy, aged 10. He strode in quickly and began work as if relieved at having something to do. He had an expression of defensive sulkiness, and was obviously on his guard. He smiled rarely, except when spoken to by a girl; then his smiling was self-conscious. He gave occasional quick, half-furtive glances over his shoulders at the other children. At closing time he threw down what he had in his hand and strode out without a word.

A.S., Boy, aged 6. He was extraordinarily self-conscious for his age, and seemed to appreciate fun and feel eager for it, but said nothing. He shook his head and used his hands rather than his voice. His excitement over trivial things was often out of proportion, while more obvious causes for amusement passed over his head unseen. The feeling he gave one was that he had a keen sense of the appropriate, was entirely occupied with his inside thoughts, and yet desired to appear to be as other children. This struggle to be as other children seemed almost a conscious effort.

J.D., Girl, aged 6. She was asked to play at school with K.S., a girl, and worker. She refused, but came to that end of the room and sat on the end of the table, where school was going on, doing a puzzle. She is very familiar with this puzzle, so it could not have absorbed more than her superficial attention, leaving most of her mind and all her emotions free to react to her immediate environment. She gave the impression of a shy, hostile animal. She flared out when K.S. pushed something rather too near her. It seems that this is the situation that she works for—to be near a pleasurable activity but not of it.

Lack of ability to play is not natural and is not an inborn characteristic; it is a neurosis, and should be reckoned as such. Children who fail in ability to play with their fellows are children with characteristics that will make them unable to combine with their fellows in after-life. Such inability is a functional disease of the emotional life—torturing in the present, and a barrier to the development of a satisfactory adult life. It is a condition that with suitable means can be cured, and a cure for it should always be sought.

CHAPTER XI

CONCLUSION

Now that the whole material for our study is before us, it is perhaps worth while for a moment to revert to the question of classification. No mind can retain for long or assimilate satisfactorily the nature of a complicated list of unrelated items. Economy of thought demands that they be divided into some sort of grouping, primarily in order that the effort of memory be diminished. Forms of play are no exception to this rule.

Before, however, a collection of facts can be divided in such a way that each item may be understood, considerable insight has to be gained into the nature and meaning of each fact. The putting of an item into a category performs a double purpose: it enables the total list to be memorised and assimilated with ease, and at the same time gives an inner meaning and purpose to the individual item.

It is essential, therefore, if the nature of play is to be grasped, that its various manifestations be divided into categories. If the categories are appropriate, the entry of each item into its place will tell us a great deal about it.

Now, play has an outer and an inner aspect: an outer aspect, which is the form which appears to the playfellow or adult observer, and an inner or psychological aspect, which is the meaning that the type of play has to the child. Classifications of play made by various observers differ according as emphasis is laid upon the outer form or the inner content. No ultimate classification will be possible which does not take into account both aspects.

The grouping here suggested shows a combination of both points of view, but with the emphasis upon the psychological content.

The standpoint from which the classification has been made is the function each form of play serves to the child who plays it. It is suggested, therefore, that there is play that expresses the bodily impulses of the child; that apperceives his environment; that prepares the child for life; that enables him to mix harmoniously with his fellows. Within each of these groupings an attempt has been made to show the existence of a number of interrelated varieties of play within the group.

Play as bodily activity is the earliest form of all children's play. During the time that speech is being acquired, play as the realisation of experience gained in previous years is the next necessity of childhood. Play as the demonstration of phantasy follows hard upon the footsteps of play as interior realisation, and interweaves all the way with it; experience feeds phantasy and phantasy interprets experience.

The child of five and six, who is learning to wield the tool of speech, and has made terms with his earlier experience, turns naturally outwards towards his environment. Play as the realisation of environment is his means of expressing his new orientation.

In and out of play as a realisation of environment goes play as a preparation for life. As early as children think of "life" at all, they may "play-train" themselves to fit into it. This form of play comes to its climax in middle school years, and with adolescence fades into reality.

No child combines naturally with its fellows before the age of four or five years; after that, delight in social play appears and grows until it reaches its maximum at about twelve to fourteen years. Group games, therefore, are considered at the end of this series, because, although many group games are played in far earlier years, yet it is the only form of children's play which is carried forward to form a major element in adult life.

Comedy and the mechanisms that determine the choice of play are common to all ages. Chapters IX and X are devoted to separate consideration of these factors.

The basis of the order of classification of the main groups of play considered is, therefore, the basis of historical growth. After four, each child *may* play all these games at any age, but the writer suggests that the peak of interest comes in the order of Chapters III to VIII. It is the particular feature of neurotic children that they may adopt any form of play at any age, and in the examples cited it is not by any means always the younger child who plays the chronologically youngest type of play. Such anomalies are characteristic of the neurotic temperament throughout life.

A classification, if it is to be true and organically interrelated, as well as logical, must also be provisional. Every classification represents the point of view from which it has been made. In a new subject at any time there may emerge new elements which may make the older classification of the subject a grouping by qualities which have now become of subsidiary rather than primary importance. When this has occurred, the classification in question should be thrown overboard and a newer one made more closely in accordance with the qualities now proved to be essential.

A classification is a finger-post, not a railway system, and in a living subject the object of a classification is to stimulate thought and to enable assimilation of the present aspects of a situation.

The classification adopted in these chapers is therefore provisional, in that little is as yet known of the *ultimate* nature of play. It is experimental, in that it has arisen out of experimental work; and it is put forward with the hope that it can be used as a practical tool by which the varieties of meaning that underlie the behaviour we speak of as " play " may be differentiated by those at work with children, and so enable a better understanding of the children we love and teach.

Play has been regarded in this book not as an accident, but as an essential function of childhood, and related in its essence to the basic qualities of mankind.

A child, as is an adult, is a creature of varied needs and activities. A child needs to learn, to eat, to excrete, and to sleep. We see here that it needs, as adults also do, to relax, to laugh, and to create; and that the problems of adaptation and understanding that oppress the adult so hardly, bear upon the child as well.

Play, when looked at from this angle, may be seen to serve four purposes:

(a) It serves as the child's means for making contact with his environment, and under this heading comes all the play considered in Chapters VI, VII, and VIII. Such play in childhood partakes of the nature of, and fulfils, much of the same social purpose as work in adult life.

(b) It makes the bridge between the child's consciousness and his emotional experience, and so fulfils the rôle that conversation, introspection, philosophy, and religion fill for the adult. In this category fall the types of play considered in Chapter IV and part of Chapter III.

(c) It represents to the child the externalised expression of his emotional life, and therefore in this aspect serves for the child the function taken by art in adult life.* Chapter V and parts of Chapter IV and some of the play described in Chapter IX describe play that fulfils this function.

(d) It serves the child as relaxation and amusement, as enjoyment and as rest, as will be seen in Chapter IX.

Play is to a child, therefore, work, thought, art, and relaxation, and cannot be pressed into any single formula. It expresses a child's relation to himself and his environment, and, without adequate opportunity for play, normal and satisfactory emotional development is not possible.

Moreover if the contention put forward on pages 113–114 is tenable, and if the author is correct in this view of play as an essential function of the passage from immaturity to emotional maturity, then any individual in whose early life these necessary opportunities for adequate play have been lacking will inevitably go on seeking them in the stuff of adult life.

Though he must do this, he will be unaware of what he is seeking. Emotional satisfactions, which the mind has missed at the period to which they properly belong, do not present themselves later in the same form. The

---

*The close relationship between play and art has been commented upon by Schiller, Groos, and Hall.

forces of destruction, aggression, and hostile emotion, which form so powerful an element for good or evil in human character, can display themselves fully in the play of childhood, and become through the expression integrated into the controlled and conscious personality. Forces unrealised in childhood remain as an inner drive forever seeking outlet, and lead men to express them not any longer in play, since this is regarded as an activity of childhood, but in industrial competition, anarchy, and war.

The less a man or a child is aware of the interior forces of his mind, the more irresistibly is he driven to express them. We have seen how fantastic is the content of much of this interior life of the mind in children: in another volume the author hopes to show how real is the logic that underlies this phantasy. The nature of this logic is, however, at utter variance with the logic of the conscious mind, and man's disharmony with himself is due to the fact that he is unaware of this situation; that, once childhood is over, he takes his games for reality, his fantastic conceptions of the world for political sanity, and his momentary myths for considered thought.

APPENDIX

(*Extract from* Una Mary: The Inner Life of a Child, *by Una Hunt*[34], *pp. 44–47*)

I WAS TAUGHT to say a prayer—"The Prayer", I called it—and for years had no idea there could be any others. It was the utterly unchristian rhyme dear to so many people from childhood associations:

> *Now I lay me down to sleep,*
> *I pray to God my soul to keep.*
> *If I should die before I wake,*
> *I pray to God my soul to take.*

. . . I felt it as a nightly terror, for the prayer is most terrifying in itself, with the suggestion of a prowling Death always ready to pounce; and the God who seems only waiting to snatch a soul away from Death is not much more reassuring. So I quaked with fear as I said it, and if I forgot a word, or coughed or sneezed in the midst of it, I was panic-stricken, and, for fear I had offended God, would hastily apologise; and, as I often had colds, my prayers were punctuated with, "I beg your pardon, God", or "I am very sorry, God; I tried not to cough" would be gasped out after I was purple in the face from trying to keep it back.

When I asked what my soul was, I was told it was part of me that I could not see, and this puzzled me greatly, for I could see all the rest of me, even my back, and the top of my head I had managed to screw a view of in the duplex mirror. I wondered what my soul could be, until one day when I was taken to a museum and saw a skeleton I found the solution. Papa told me it was the inside framework of a man, the part of him that was left after he died. The Boned Man I called it at first, and then, when I heard there was one inside me, too, I knew, of course, that must be the soul, the part I asked God to keep.

Before this I had thought of Death as a sort of purple-black ghost with long-reaching arms, like the huge shadows that waved across my ceiling when the gas flickered in the wind at night. Often I have lain, almost paralysed with terror, watching them with awful fascination until I could bear it no longer, and would shout that I wanted a drink of water; for as soon as someone came into the room the terror seemed to go, and they were just ordinary shadows again. Sometimes I heard the far-off whistle of a train, and that, too, seemed to make the shadows normal at once. How I used to strain my ears for a train! . . .

After I saw the skeleton, Death became even more awful, able to slip one's flesh off one's bones and leave the soul "naked and white". I had heard Lizzie apply those adjectives to the soul, and they were certainly an accurate description of a skeleton.

I felt, as I said "The Prayer" before going to bed, that Death was more than likely to appear during the night—"The Prayer" gave no hint of his being able to come in the daytime—so each night I was careful, as soon as I had taken off my stockings—I kept them on while I said my prayers—to scramble into bed as quickly as possible in order to hide my bare feet under the bedclothes and so prevent Death's catching hold of them. I had gotten the idea that he could not lay hold of my skeleton through clothes but had to find a spot of bare skin to begin on, and if he once got hold of even a single toe I was sure one pull would be enough—out would come my bones, leaving my body turned inside out like an empty glove.

REFERENCES

1. Mead, M. (1930) *Growing Up in New Guinea*. New York: Morrow. (London: Kegan Paul, 1931.)
2. LoBagola, B. K. A. I. (1930) *LoBagola: an African Savage's Own Story*. New York: Knopf; London: Allen & Unwin.
3. Byng, D. (1932) *The Byng Ballads*. London: John Lane, Bodley Head.
4. Maeterlinck, M. (1909) *The Bluebird*. London: Methuen.
5. Grahame, K. (1908) *The Wind in the Willows*. London: Methuen.
6. Herbert, A. P. (1930) *The Water Gipsies*. London: Methuen.
7. Marshall, H. (1931) 'Children's play, games and amusements.' *In:* Murchison, C. (Ed.) *A Handbook of Child Psychology.* London: Oxford University Press; Worcester, MA: Clark University Press.
8. Froebel, F. (1912) *Chief Writings on Education.* (Translated by Fletcher, S. S. F., Welton, J.) London: Arnold.
9. Spencer, H. (1855) 'Aesthetic sentiment.' *In: The Principles of Psychology, Vol. II.* London. (p. 693.)
10. Grasberger, L. (1864) *Erziehung und Unterricht im klassischen Alterthum, Vol. I.* Würzburg: Stahel.
11. Groos, K. (1898) *The Play of Animals.* (Translated by Baldwin, E. L.) London: Chapman & Hall; New York: Appleton.
12. Groos, K. (1901) *The Play of Man.* (Translated by Baldwin, E. L.) London: Heinemann; New York: Appleton.
13. Hall, G. S., and pupils (1907) *Aspects of Child Life and Education.* London and Boston: Ginn & Co.
14. Hall, G. S., and pupils (1921) *Youth: its Education, Regimen and Hygiene.* London and New York: Appleton.
15. Sully, J. (1896) *Studies of Childhood.* London and New York: Appleton.
16. Freud, S. (1922) *Beyond the Pleasure Principle.* (Translated by Hubback, C. J. M.) London and Vienna: International Psychoanalytical Press.
17. Isaacs, S. (1930) *Intellectual Growth in Young Children.* London: Routledge; New York: Harcourt Brace.
18. Stern, W. (1924) *Psychology of Early Childhood: up to the Sixth Year of Age.* (Translated by Barwell, A.) London: Allen; New York: Holt.
19. Froebel, F. (1895) *Pedagogics of the Kindergarten.* (Translated by Jarvis, J.) London: Appleton.
20. Bühler, C. (1933) 'The child and its activity with practical material.' *British Journal of Educational Psychology*, **3**, 27–41.
21. Swift, E. J. (1918) *Psychology and the Day's Work: a Study in the Application of Psychology to Daily Life.* London: Allen & Unwin.

22. Bühler, C. (1935) *From Birth to Maturity.* London: Kegan Paul.
23. Bühler, C. (1930) *The First Year of Life.* (Translated by Greenberg, P., Ripin, R.) New York: John Day.
24. Russell, pupils of B. and M. (1934) *Thinking in Front of Yourself.* London: Janus Press.
25. Milne, A. A. (1926) *Winnie the Pooh.* London: Methuen.
26. Bühler, C. (1928) *Kindheit und Jugend. Genese des Bewusstseins.* Psychologische Monographien, Vol. III. Leipzig: Herzel.
27. Wallon, H. (1933) *Les Origines du Caractère chez l'Enfant.* Paris: Boivin.
28. Bridges, K. B. (1931) *Social and Emotional Development of the Pre-school Child.* London: Kegan Paul.
29. Ernst, O. (1913) *Roswitha's Day.* (Translated by Caton, A. C.) London: A. C. Caton.
30. Ernst, O. (1914) *Roswitha or Philosophy?* (Translated by Caton, A. C.) London: A. C. Caton.
31. Isaacs, S. (1933) *Social Development in Young Children. A Study of Beginnings.* London: Routledge; New York: Harcourt Brace.
32. Piaget, J. (1926) *The Language and Thought of the Child.* (Translated by Warden, M.) London: Kegan Paul; New York: Harcourt Brace.
33. Collingwood, R. G. (1933) *An Essay on Philosophical Method.* Oxford: Clarendon Press.
34. Hunt, U. (1917) *Una Mary: the Inner Life of a Child.* New York: Scribner's.
35. Piaget, J. (1929) *The Child's Conception of the World.* (Translated by Tomlinson, J. and Tomlinson, A.) London: Kegan Paul; New York: Harcourt Brace.
36. Thorburn, M. (1933) *Edward and Marigold.* London: Allen & Unwin.
37. Drummond, M. (1921) *Five Years Old or Thereabouts.* London: Arnold.
38. Froebel, F. (1906) *Education of Man.* (Translated by Hailmann, W. N.) London: Appleton.
39. Nunn, P. T. (1922) *Education: its Data and First Principles.* London: Arnold.
40. Cook, H. C. (1917) *The Play Way. An Essay in Educational Method.* London: Heinemann.
41. Roth, W. E. (1902) *Games, Sports and Amusements. North Queensland Ethnography Bulletin, No. 4.* Brisbane: Vaughan.
42. Culin, R. S. (1895) *Korean Games.* Philadelphia: University of Pennsylvania.
43. Hetzer, H. (1927) *Das volkstümliche Kinderspiel.* Vienna: Deutscher Verlag für Jugend und Volk.
44. Bergson, H. (1911) *Le Rire. Essai sur la Signification du Comique.* 7ᵐᵉ Edn. Paris: Alcan.
45. Murray, E. R. (1914) *Froebel as a Pioneer in Modern Psychology.* London: George Philip.
46. Sully, J. (1902) *An Essay on Laughter.* London: Longmans Green.
47. Bairnsfather, B. (1919) *From Mud to Mufti; with Old Bill on All Fronts.* London: Richards.
48. Greig, J. Y. T. (1923) *The Psychology of Laughter and Comedy.* London: Allen & Unwin.
49. Du Maurier, D. (1934) *Gerald, a Portrait.* London: Gollancz.
50. Smith, T. L. (1907) *In:* Hall, G. S., and pupils *Aspects of Child Life and Education.* London and Boston: Ginn & Co.

51. Bühler, C. (1931) 'The social behaviour of the child.' *In:* Murchison, C. (Ed.) *A Handbook of Child Psychology.* London: Oxford University Press; Worcester, MA: Clark University Press.
52. Hollingworth, L. S. (1926) *Gifted Children: their Nature and Nurture.* New York: Macmillan.
53. Winkler-Hermaden, V. (1927) *Zur Psychologie des Jugendführers. Quellen und Studien zum Jugendkunde, Nr. 6.* Jena: Fischer.

INDEX

ADDENDUM

THE DR MARGARET LOWENFELD TRUST

W HEN DR LOWENFELD DIED in 1973, two small trusts, amalgamated in 1983 to form the Dr Margaret Lowenfeld Trust, were set up to perpetuate her ideas and methods and to keep practice based on them up to date. Since its foundation, the Trust has supported a Margaret Lowenfeld Research Fellow (currently Dr Cathy Urwin) in the Child Care and Development Group at the University of Cambridge. It has helped with the publication of Lowenfeld's *The World Technique* and a collection of her selected papers under the title *Child Psychotherapy, War and the Normal Child,* edited by Cathy Urwin and John Hood-Williams. The Trustees have also supported other research by former Institute of Child Psychology students, and have fostered the growing interest in Lowenfeld's methods in the United Kingdom and in the United States of America. An annual Lowenfeld Seminar on child psychotherapy is held in Cambridge, with a mixed programme bringing together researchers and practitioners with an interest in relations between emotionality and non-verbal thought.

The Dr Margaret Lowenfeld Trust is a charitable body that has already achieved much, and would do more were resources not so limited. Information about the Trust, Dr Lowenfeld's work and the availability of the methods and publications may be had from:

Dr Martin Richards, Child Care and Development Group, Free School Lane, Cambridge CB2 3RF

or from the Chairman of the Trustees, Dr H. Beric Wright, Brudenell House, Quainton, Aylesbury, Bucks HP22 4AW.